Medical Billing & Coding

2023-2024

- 📓 **Note-Taking Techniques:** Discover various methods for taking effective and organized notes during lectures or while reading textbooks.
- 💬**Critical Thinking Skills:** Develop your ability to analyze, evaluate, and synthesize information to make informed decisions and solve problems.
- ⏰ **Time Blocking and the Pomodoro Technique:** Learn about time management techniques like time blocking and the Pomodoro Technique to enhance productivity
- 🏆 **Stress Relief Strategies:** Overcome exam anxiety with mindfulness, relaxation exercises, and mental resilience techniques.
- ⬛ **Practice Makes Perfect:** Explore the importance of practice exams, sample questions, and mock tests, and understand how to analyze your performance to identify areas for improvement.
- ⚫ **Test-Taking Tactics:** Master the art of answering different types of questions, managing your time during the exam, and maintaining focus under pressure.

The following is a disclaimer of liability:

The goal of this book is to provide the reader with background information on the numerous topics that are discussed throughout the book. It is offered for sale with the understanding that neither the author nor the publisher are engaged in the practice of providing professional advice of any type, including but not limited to advice pertaining to legal matters, medical matters, or other matters. In the event that one need the aid of a professional, one must seek the assistance of an experienced professional who is qualified to provide it.

This book has been laboriously labored over in an effort to make it as accurate as is humanly feasible, and it has taken a lot of labor. However, there is a possibility that there are inaccuracies, both in the typography and the actual content of the article. The author and publisher of this book do not accept any responsibility or liability to any third party for any loss or damage caused, or represented to have been caused, directly or indirectly, by the information that is included in this book. This rule applies to any loss or harm that may have been caused, or is suspected of having been caused, by the information that is presented in this book.

This information is provided "as is," without any guarantees or warranties regarding its completeness, accuracy, usefulness, or timeliness. The information is presented "as is" without any guarantees or warranties of any kind. The reader is highly encouraged to seek the opinion of a certified expert or professionals in the field in order to obtain the most up-to-date knowledge that is currently available.

information and compiled data.

In no way, shape, or form does the viewpoints or policies of any specific organisation or professional body come over in this book in any kind whatsoever. Any slights that could be interpreted as being directed toward specific individuals or groups were not intended, despite the fact that they may have occurred.

TABLE OF CONTENT

STUDY GUIDE

Chapter 1: Introduction to Medical Billing and Coding
1.1 The Importance of Medical Billing and Coding
1.2 The Role of Medical Billers and Coders
1.3 Recent Trends in Healthcare

Chapter 2: The Healthcare Industry Today
2.1 Understanding Healthcare Providers
2.2 Insurance Providers and Payers
2.3 Regulatory Bodies and Compliance

Chapter 3: Medical Terminology
3.1 Anatomy and Physiology
3.2 Common Medical Abbreviations
3.3 Disease and Medical Condition Terminology

Chapter 4: Medical Coding
4.1 Introduction to Medical Coding
4.2 ICD-10-CM (International Classification of Diseases, 10th Edition, Clinical Modification)
4.3 CPT (Current Procedural Terminology)
4.4 HCPCS (Healthcare Common Procedure Coding System)
4.5 Modifiers in Coding

Chapter 5: Medical Billing
5.1 The Basics of Medical Billing
5.2 The Claims Process
5.3 Billing Software and Technology
5.4 Reimbursement Methods

Chapter 6: Compliance and Regulations
6.1 HIPAA (Health Insurance Portability and Accountability Act)
6.2 Fraud and Abuse Regulations
6.3 EHR (Electronic Health Records) and Meaningful Use
6.4 Updates for 2023-2024

Chapter 7: Electronic Health Records (EHR)
7.1 EHR Implementation
7.2 Benefits and Challenges
7.3 EHR and Billing Integration

Chapter 8: Reimbursement Methods
8.1 Fee-for-Service vs. Value-Based Care
8.2 Medicare and Medicaid
8.3 Commercial Insurance
8.4 Accountable Care Organizations (ACOs)

Chapter 9: Auditing and Quality Assurance
9.1 The Role of Auditing in Healthcare
9.2 Quality Assurance and Compliance Audits
9.3 Preparing for an Audit

Chapter 10: Emerging Trends in Medical Billing and Coding
10.1 Telehealth and Remote Coding
10.2 Artificial Intelligence in Medical Coding
10.3 Telemedicine Regulations and Reimbursement

Chapter 11: Career Development and Certification
11.1 Preparing for Certification
11.2 Continuing Education
11.3 Job Opportunities and Career Growth

Chapter 12: The Future of Medical Billing and Coding
12.1 Anticipated Changes in Healthcare
12.2 The Impact of Healthcare Reform
12.3 Preparing for 2024 and Beyond

Chapter 13: Telehealth Billing
13.1 Telehealth Services and Reimbursement
13.2 Telehealth Coding Guidelines
13.3 Telehealth Billing Challenges and Solutions

Chapter 14: Revenue Cycle Management

14.1 Introduction to Revenue Cycle Management (RCM)

14.2 Key Stages of RCM

14.3 Best Practices for Optimizing RCM

Chapter 15: Denials Management

15.1 Common Reasons for Claim Denials

15.2 Denials Resolution Strategies

15.3 Reducing Denials through Improved Documentation

Chapter 16: Medical Billing and Coding in Specialties

16.1 Coding and Billing for Cardiology

16.2 Obstetrics and Gynecology Billing

16.3 Orthopedic Surgery Coding

16.4 Mental Health and Behavioral Health Coding

Chapter 17: Legal and Ethical Considerations

17.1 Legal Issues in Medical Billing and Coding

17.2 Ethical Dilemmas and Decision-Making

17.3 Patient Privacy and Confidentiality

Chapter 18: International Classification of Diseases (ICD) Updates

18.1 ICD-11: An Overview

18.2 Preparing for the Transition to ICD-11

18.3 Impact of ICD-11 on Medical Billing and Coding

Introduction to Medical Coding and Billing is Covered in Chapter 1.

In the constantly shifting landscape of the healthcare industry, where the care of patients is the primary focus, the procedures that take place behind the scenes to ensure that medical services are appropriately documented, invoiced, and reimbursed play an essential role. Billing and coding for medical services are two interrelated fields that are necessary to make this procedure possible. This chapter digs into the fundamental building blocks of medical billing and coding, their significance in the healthcare industry, as well as their progression throughout the course of time.

1.1 The Significance of Billing and Coding in the Medical Industry

1.1.1 The System of Healthcare Provision and Delivery

Imagine a busy private practice or a busy hospital where a variety of healthcare providers, including doctors, nurses, and other allied health professionals, are dedicated to diagnosing and treating patients. In this fast-paced and high-pressure atmosphere, the primary concentration is placed on the care, diagnosis, and treatment of individual patients. However, the ecosystem of healthcare is significantly more complicated, and it consists of a large number of moving pieces that must cooperate in order to deliver care that is both effective and efficient.

1.1.2 The Nexus of the Financial System

Medical billing and coding are the activities that sit at the epicenter of this ecosystem's financial structure. These two professions are like the unseen builders of the healthcare business; they put in a lot of hard work to make sure that those who offer medical care get paid fairly for their efforts. The following are some of the reasons why medical billing and coding are so important:

Producing Money or Revenue

The generation of money for healthcare organizations is an essential part of the function that is performed by medical billing and coding. Following the provision of healthcare services, these services need to be interpreted into standardized codes, invoiced to insurance companies, government programs, or individual patients, and payments must subsequently be collected. Coding and billing that is accurate are absolutely necessary in order to guarantee that medical professionals are paid a reasonable amount for the services they render.

Compliance with Regulations

The healthcare industry is subject to stringent regulations, and failure to comply with these regulations can have severe repercussions, including possible legal action and financial penalties. Professionals who work in medical billing and coding play an essential part in ensuring that healthcare institutions comply with requirements concerning billing and documentation. The Health Insurance Portability and Accountability Act (HIPAA), as well as coding requirements and government reimbursement mechanisms, are all part of this.

Care and Maintenance of Patient Records

Maintaining patient records that are complete and accurate requires accurate medical coding as a foundational component. Not only do these records provide a historical narrative of a patient's journey through the healthcare system, but they also assist in the process of making educated medical decisions. When conducting diagnostic evaluations and formulating treatment strategies for patients, medical professionals need access to accurate patient data in order to arrive at accurate diagnoses.

Claims Made on Insurance

Professionals that specialize in medical billing and coding are tasked with the responsibility of drafting and submitting insurance claims on behalf of healthcare providers. This process can be difficult due to the fact that many insurance providers have their own set of regulations and prerequisites. Coding and billing that is accurate increases the likelihood that insurance claims will be processed swiftly and that payments will be received on time.

Manage Your Expenses

Controlling costs is an essential component of healthcare, both for individual patients and for the organizations that provide healthcare. Patients should not be charged more than necessary, and healthcare organizations should be able to effectively manage the revenue they bring in thanks to accurate billing. Errors in coding and billing can result in lost money and legal conflicts, making accuracy a vital component of effective cost management.

1.1.3 Interaction Between Patient and Provider

Although medical billing and coding are mostly done behind the scenes, they have a direct influence on the interactions that take place between patients and their providers. Coding and billing that is accurate leads to financial dealings that are both honest and open between patients and the healthcare providers that treat them. It is important for patients to have an understanding of both their medical costs and their insurance claims in order to create trust in the healthcare system.

1.1.4 Uninterrupted Development

The ever-increasing scale of the healthcare sector places an even greater emphasis on the significance of accurate medical billing and coding. For instance, healthcare spending in the United States has been steadily climbing for the past many years, and in 2019, it reached a total of $3.8 trillion. As medical care continues to advance, there is likely to be an increased demand for qualified experts in the fields of medical billing and coding, which will result in the creation of a wide variety of job openings.

1.2 The Importance of Medical Billers and Coders in the Healthcare Industry

1.2.1 Coders in the Medical Field

Coders in the medical field act as translators between patients and the healthcare industry. They do this by ascribing standardized codes to the diagnoses, procedures, and services that healthcare providers give to patients. The purposes of billing, filing insurance claims, and doing statistical analysis all make use of these codes. Coders in the medical industry make certain that each and every facet of a patient's interaction with the healthcare system is accurately documented and reflected by a corresponding code.

Different kinds of codes

ICD-10-CM stands for the International Classification of Diseases, 10th Edition, Clinical Modification. This classification system is utilized for the purpose of assigning codes to diseases, disorders, and symptoms.

CPT stands for "Current Procedural Terminology," and it's the terminology that's used to code medical operations and services.

HCPCS stands for "Healthcare Common Procedure Coding System," and it's the system that's used to code services, supplies, and equipment that aren't covered by CPT codes.

1.2.2 Medical Billing Professionals

Medical coders are responsible for assigning codes, while medical billers are responsible for converting those codes into claims. Depending on the source of payment, these claims are either sent to insurance companies, healthcare programs run by the government, or individual individuals. Because mistakes in claims can result in payment delays and disputes, the work of a medical biller requires painstaking attention to detail at every stage of the process.

The Methods Used in Billing

Registration of the Patient: The first step in the process is when the patient registers themselves at a medical facility. Information concerning the patient's demographics and insurance coverage is gathered.

Coding is the process in which medical coders examine a patient's medical records in order to assign appropriate codes to diagnoses, procedures, and services.

Billing requires medical billers to use the coded information to build claims, which are then sent to the appropriate parties for payment consideration.

Posting of Payments: As soon as billers receive payments, they immediately post them to the patient's account and verify that the payments correspond to the claims.

Follow-Up: In order to settle payment issues and make certain that claims are processed in a timely way, billers frequently engage in activities that fall under the category of "follow-up."

1.2.3 The Specifics of the Role

Accuracy and Observance of Regulations

Coders and billers in the medical industry are required to follow specific criteria for coding and billing, which ensures that patients are charged fairly for the services received. The observance of laws and policies, such as the HIPAA, is of the utmost significance.

Competence in technological matters

Medical coders and billers need to be adept in the use of electronic health records (EHR) and billing software as the healthcare business grows more dependent on technology. These technologies make the process of coding and billing easier, which ultimately results in increased productivity.

Exchange of information

Professionals in the fields of medical billing and coding frequently engage with patients, as well as healthcare providers and insurance organizations. When it comes to resolving issues, gaining clarity on codes, and ensuring that billing processes go smoothly, effective communication is absolutely necessary.

Resolution of Issues

Coding and billing can be extremely difficult tasks, and individuals who work in these jobs frequently face obstacles such as claim denials or coding anomalies. For the purpose of resolving these challenges, problem-solving skills are absolutely necessary.

1.2.4 Different Career Options

Coding and billing in the medical industry both provide a variety of career routes, making them approachable for people of varying interests and levels of expertise. The following are examples of some of the more prevalent jobs in this sector:

Coders in the medical field are the ones who are in charge of assigning codes to diagnoses and procedures.

As a medical biller, your primary responsibilities will include the production and filing of claims as well as the processing of payments.

An auditor of medical coding verifies the correctness and legality of the coding.

The Health Information Technician is responsible for managing the data associated with health information, including coding and recording.

A practice manager is responsible for overseeing all administrative tasks inside a healthcare facility, including billing and coding.

1.3 Emerging Patterns in the Healthcare Industry

1.3.1 The Development of New Technologies

The field of medicine is currently experiencing a period of rapid technological advancement. Electronic health records, also known as EHRs, have supplanted paper records as the preferred method of documenting patient information because of their seamless integration with the coding and billing procedures. Telehealth and telemedicine have also seen substantial growth in popularity in recent years. These fields provide remote medical treatments, which call for advanced knowledge of medical coding and invoicing.

1.3.2 Amendments to the Regulations

The regulations governing the healthcare industry are often being updated, which can have substantial effects on medical billing and coding. The implementation of ICD-10 in 2015 was a significant shift, and subsequent revisions are anticipated. In addition, the proliferation of value-based care and alternative payment models is redefining the manner in which healthcare services are compensated, making it necessary for professionals working in billing and coding to adjust their practices.

1.3.3 Analyses of the Data

The analysis of patient data is becoming an increasingly vital part of the healthcare industry. Organizations are able to spot trends, improve patient care, and boost billing and coding accuracy when they analyze huge volumes of data pertaining to the healthcare industry. Decision-making in the healthcare industry that is informed by data analysis is becoming increasingly common.

1.3.4 Remote Coding and Telehealth Services

The COVID-19 pandemic sped up the adoption of telehealth, which led to a rise in the demand for specialists who are familiar with the one-of-a-kind coding and billing problems that are linked with remote healthcare services. Coding and invoicing for telehealth services require specialized understanding to guarantee that patients are properly reimbursed for their virtual encounters.

1.3.5 Application of Artificial Intelligence to the Coding of Medical Records

The use of artificial intelligence (AI) is beginning to penetrate the medical coding industry. The medical records of a patient can be reviewed by AI algorithms, which can then extract pertinent information and suggest appropriate codes. Despite the fact that AI has the potential to improve productivity, it still needs human oversight in order to guarantee accuracy and comply with regulations.

The Current State of the Healthcare Industry in Chapter 2

The business of providing medical care is a huge and intricate ecosystem that includes a diverse group of stakeholders, services, and organizational structures. It is essential for anyone participating in the healthcare business or aspiring to be a part of the industry, especially those who work in medical billing and coding, to have a solid understanding of the present state of the industry. In this chapter, we will investigate the many facets of the healthcare business in 2023-2024, ranging from the most important actors to the transforming models of care and the influence of recent local and international occurrences.

2.1 Recognizing the Roles of Healthcare Providers

The healthcare business is made up of a broad group of providers, each of which provides patients with a unique set of services and plays an important part in the overall process of providing healthcare. These service providers can be placed into the following categories on a more general level:

2.1.1 Medical Centers and Hospitals

Hospitals are the primary establishments for the provision of medical care because of the extensive array of services they provide, which range from first aid and surgery to specialized medical care. In the years 2023 and 2024, hospitals will continue to develop in order to better serve the ever-evolving requirements of their patients. The following are key trends in hospital care:

Care That Is More Tailored Numerous healthcare facilities are currently in the process of establishing specialized centers of excellence that will concentrate on fields such as oncology, cardiology, and orthopedics. Patients can receive care that is extremely specialized and cutting-edge at these facilities.

Integration of Telehealth Services Hospitals are progressively embracing telehealth services in order to provide remote consultations and follow-up care for patients. In recent years, particularly during the COVID-19 pandemic, telemedicine has emerged as an extremely useful tool.

Initiatives for Population Health Hospitals are becoming more proactive in their approach to population health by implementing wellness programs, preventative care, and initiatives for population health management.

2.1.2 Primary Care Providers (also known as PCPs)

Patients who are interested in receiving medical treatment should get in touch with a primary care provider first. Primary care physicians include family doctors, internists, and pediatricians. Over the course of the past few years, primary care has experienced a number of shifts, including:

Patient-Centered Medical Homes (PCMHs): The PCMH concept focuses on improving patient care by increasing access to primary care services and care coordination. PCMHs are also known as medical homes. The function of primary care within the healthcare system is strengthened by this paradigm.

Telehealth services have improved access to primary care, making it easier for patients to interact with their primary care clinicians remotely. This application of telemedicine is known as "primary care telemedicine."

2.1.3 Centers for Outpatient Ambulatory Care

Ambulatory care centers, which also include urgent care clinics and outpatient surgical centers, are facilities that offer a wide variety of outpatient medical services. They provide alternatives to hospital-based care that are more convenient and less expensive. The following are some current trends in ambulatory care:

Care at Your Convenience Ambulatory care clinics are increasingly putting an emphasis on delivering care that is both convenient and accessible. This typically includes offering extended hours and same-day appointments.

Clinics Specializing in Particular disorders A growing number of ambulatory care facilities are creating clinics that specialize in treating particular disorders, such as clinics for the treatment of wounds and clinics for the management of pain.

Retail Clinics: Retail clinics can be found in pharmacies and other stores, and they provide fundamental medical services such as immunizations and minor acute treatment. This makes healthcare even more accessible to the general public.

2.1.4 Centers for Long-Term Medical Care

Long-term care facilities, such as nursing homes and assisted living facilities, are an essential component of the healthcare system for geriatric patients and people living with long-term diseases. Long-term care has undergone transformations in recent years as a direct result of the growing elderly population.

Care That Is Centered on the Person Increasingly, long-term care institutions are adopting patient-centered care models, which put the residents' specific preferences and requirements at the forefront of treatment decisions.

Home and Community-Based Services (HCBS): There is an increasing emphasis on the provision of long-term care services in home and community settings, which allows individuals to age in place. This enables individuals to maintain their independence for as long as possible.

2.1.5 Providers Specializing in Specialized Care

Providers of specialized care are an essential component of the healthcare ecosystem. In addition to primary care, hospitals, and facilities for long-term care, specialized care providers are essential. These service providers are as follows:

Providers of Mental Health and Behavioral Health: The significance of mental health services has recently come to be acknowledged, which has led to a rise in the integration of mental health services into primary care and a wider availability of these services.

Centers for Rehabilitation: As the population as a whole ages, there will be an increased demand for rehabilitation services such as occupational therapy and physical therapy offered in rehabilitation centers.

These types of care offer patients and their families compassionate end-of-life care and support services. Hospice and palliative care are two examples of these kind of services.

Providers of Dental and Vision Care It is widely acknowledged that oral and vision health are critical components of total health, which has led to a growing integration of dental and vision care with medical treatment.

2.2 Insurance Companies and Their Customers

Because it enables patients to better handle the expenditures associated with medical care, health insurance is an essential component of the healthcare business. The following are some categories that can be used to classify insurance providers and payers:

2.2.1 Individual or Family Health Insurance Coverage

Individuals and corporations can choose from a number of health plans made available by private health insurance firms. The following are some key trends in private health insurance:

Increasingly, insurance companies are making their plans more adaptable so that they can better serve the particular requirements of both individuals and corporations.

Services Digitales: Numerous private insurance companies are working to improve their digital services, which will enable their members to access their insurance information and resources online.

Wellness and Prevention Programs: Insurance companies are putting an emphasis on wellness and prevention programs in an effort to promote healthy lifestyles and cut down on the expense of medical care.

2.2.2 Health Care Programs Offered by the Government

A key part of ensuring that certain groups of people have access to medical care is played by the provision of insurance by the government in the form of programs like Medicare and Medicaid in the United States. Recent changes made by the government to its healthcare programs include the following:

Increased Access to Healthcare Services As a result of Medicaid Expansion, a number of states have made it possible for more low-income people to participate in their respective Medicaid programs.

Plans Under Medicare Advantage: Medicare Advantage plans, which are provided by private insurers and are gaining in popularity as a result of the additional benefits they give in comparison to standard Medicare, are known as Medicare Advantage plans.

Value-Based Payment Models: More and more government programs are beginning to use value-based payment models, which relate reimbursement to the quality of care that is provided.

2.2.3 Organizations Managing Patient Care

Intermediaries that enter into contractual agreements with healthcare providers in order to administer and coordinate patient care are known as managed care organizations. These organizations include Health Maintenance Organizations (HMOs) and Preferred Provider Organizations (PPOs). Some current trends in managed care are as follows:

Care Coordination as the Primary Focus Managed care organizations are placing a primary emphasis on care coordination as the primary focus of their efforts to improve the overall quality and effectiveness of care.

Integration of Telehealth Many managed care companies now cover telehealth services, which broadens patients' access to care provided virtually.

Patient Engagement To assist individuals in making educated decisions regarding their healthcare, managed care organizations place a high priority on activities that encourage patient participation and education.

2.3 Organizations Responsible for Regulation and Compliance

In order to protect patients and maintain high standards of care, the healthcare business is subject to a myriad of regulations and forms of control. The following will be important regulatory agencies and compliance considerations in 2023-2024:

2.3.1 The Department of Health and Human Services

Many facets of healthcare, such as Medicare and Medicaid, fall under the purview of the Department of Health and Human Services (HHS) of the United States of America. The Department of Health and Human Services is an essential participant in the formulation and execution of healthcare policy.

2.3.2 The Centers for Medicare & Medicaid Services (often known as CMS)

The Centers for Medicare & Medicaid Services (CMS) is the federal agency that is in charge of administering the nation's primary healthcare programs, such as Medicare and Medicaid. It is also responsible for regulating healthcare providers, establishing reimbursement rates, and promoting value-based care models.

2.3.3 The Commission of Joint Affairs

Accrediting and certifying healthcare organizations and programs in the United States is the objective of the non-profit organization known as the Joint Commission. The Joint Commission accreditation is an important marker of both quality and safety in the healthcare industry.

2.3.4 HIPAA, or the Health Insurance Portability and Accountability Act

The Health Insurance Portability and Accountability Act of 1996, also known as HIPAA, is a federal law that ensures the confidentiality of medical records of patients. To ensure the security of patient information, it is essential for healthcare providers, insurers, and others working in medical billing and coding to comply with the HIPAA requirements.

2.3.5 Coding Guidelines for the ICD-10-CM and the CPT

Both the International Classification of Diseases, 10th Edition, Clinical Modification (ICD-10-CM) and the Current Procedural Terminology (CPT) are continuously subject to changes and adjustments. Coders and billing specialists in the medical field are required to maintain current knowledge of these coding principles in order to guarantee compliance.

2.3.6 Value-Based Care and Quality Reporting in Healthcare

Value-based care models, in which remuneration is related to the quality of care provided, are becoming increasingly prevalent in the healthcare business, which is changing in this direction. It is absolutely necessary to ensure compliance with quality reporting measures in order to receive the best possible reimbursement.

2.4 Emerging Patterns in the Healthcare Industry

Not only is it essential to have a grasp of the major actors and regulatory agencies in the healthcare business, but it is also essential to be aware of the most recent trends and advancements that are influencing the industry in 2023-2024:

2.4.1 Remote Medical Services, Also Known as Telehealth

As a result of the COVID-19 epidemic, telehealth and telemedicine have witnessed substantial expansion and acceptance in recent years. These technological advancements have resulted in an increase in access to medical care as well as a transformation in the delivery of medical services.

2.4.2 Applications of Artificial Intelligence (AI) in the Healthcare Industry

There are many different uses for AI in the healthcare industry, ranging from providing diagnostic help to anticipating disease outbreaks. Artificial intelligence is helping to automate code assignment in the medical coding industry, which is boosting accuracy.

2.4.3 Care that Is Centered on Values

The movement toward value-based care models, which put a higher emphasis on patient outcomes and the quality of care, is altering the delivery of healthcare services as well as the methods by which they are reimbursed.

2.4.4 Health Information Exchange (often abbreviated as "HIE")

The ability of healthcare practitioners to safely communicate patient data through the use of health information exchange improves care coordination while also cutting down on unnecessary testing and procedures.

2.4.5 Accurate Medicine and Treatment

The practice of medicine that is individualized to the specific qualities of each patient is known as "precision medicine." Diagnostics and treatment options are being improved as a result of this technique.

2.4.6 Analyses of Data in the Healthcare Sector

The use of data analytics in healthcare is becoming increasingly vital for spotting trends, bettering the results for patients, and raising the accuracy of billing and coding.

2.4.7 The Readiness of the Public Health System

The COVID-19 pandemic brought to light the significance of public health preparedness and response, leading to increased investment in pandemic planning and management by governments and healthcare institutions.

The Terminology of Medicine, Chapter 3

The language of medicine is known as medical terminology, and it plays an important role in the healthcare industry by promoting clear communication among medical personnel, accurate record keeping of patients, and precise medical coding and invoicing. In this chapter, we will discuss the principles of medical terminology, the components of medical terms, and the significance of having a strong understanding of medical language in the context of the healthcare industry in 2023-2024.

3.1 The Importance of Terminology in the Medical Field

3.1.1 A Language Spoken Everywhere

The terminology used in medicine is a kind of international language that is spoken by people working in healthcare all around the world. It is able to traverse linguistic and cultural barriers, ensuring that a medical phrase or condition is interpreted in the same manner regardless of the healthcare context in which it is encountered.

3.1.2 Accuracy and Unmistakability

Clarity in healthcare communication can be achieved by the use of accurate medical terminology. When those working in healthcare employ standardized vocabulary, there is very little possibility for ambiguity or misinterpretation of what is being communicated.

3.1.3 Documentation That Is Accurate

When it comes to documenting patient information and medical procedures, having accurate medical language is absolutely necessary. Standardized terminologies are essential to the efficient organization and storage of patient data in electronic health records, often known as EHRs.

3.1.4 Coding and Billing in the Medical Industry

A comprehensive understanding of medical language is absolutely necessary in the field of medical billing and coding. Coders make use of medical jargon in order to assign precise codes to diagnoses and procedures. In doing so, they ensure that medical professionals are reimbursed in an acceptable manner.

3.2 The Fundamental Concepts Underlying Medical Terminology

The vocabulary used in medicine frequently appears to be difficult to understand due to the use of lengthy terms and technical jargon. On the other hand, it is built up from a number of essential components, which allows more people to access it and makes it simpler to comprehend.

3.2.1 The Origins of Words

The essential component of a medical term is referred to as the word root, which is sometimes referred to as the foundation word. It offers the most fundamental interpretation of the term. For instance, the prefix "cardi-" refers to the organ known as the heart. It is from this root that a number of medical terminology pertaining to the heart, such as "cardiology" (the study of the heart) and "cardiologist" (a doctor who specializes in heart care), are derived.

3.2.2 The Use of Prefixes

The meaning of a word can be altered by attaching a prefix to the beginning of the word. They frequently denote a location, a time, a number, or one of several other characteristics. For instance, the prefix "pre-" means "before," and the term "preoperative" refers to actions or circumstances that take place before a surgical operation.

3.2.3 Adding on a Suffix

Suffixes are affixes that are added to the end of a word in order to change the meaning of the term. Suffixes often indicate a condition, treatment, or disease. For example, the suffix "-ectomy" can signify "removal" or "excision," and the term "appendectomy" describes the process of surgically removing the appendix from the body.

3.2.4 Forms That Combine Together

Combining forms are produced by combining the root of a word with a vowel, most commonly the letter "o." The process of combining roots with prefixes and suffixes is simplified by using this form. For instance, the word root "gastr-" (which refers to the stomach) can be joined with the vowel "o" to get "gastro-," which is then used in terms such as "gastroscopy" (which refers to an examination of the stomach) and "gastrointestinal" (which refers to the stomach and the intestines).

3.2.5 Prefixes and Suffixes Used Commonly in Medical Terminology

It is helpful to become familiar with some frequent prefixes and suffixes in order to comprehend medical terminology. These prefixes and suffixes are as follows:

Various Prefixes:

"A-" or "An-": Without or absence of (for example, "anemia" refers to a deficiency in red blood cells).

"Dys-" means "difficult" or "painful." For example, "dyspnea" means "breathing that is difficult or painful."

The prefix "hypo-" means "below" or "insufficient" (for example, "hypoglycemia" means "low blood sugar").

The prefix "poly-" means "many" or "much." For example, "polyuria" refers to profuse urinating.

Adding a Suffix:

The suffix "-itis" denotes inflammation; for example, "tonsillitis" refers to inflammation of the tonsils.

"-ology" refers to the study of a particular topic (for example, "cardiology" is the study of the cardiovascular system).

"-ectomy" refers to a surgical procedure that removes something (for example, "appendectomy" refers to the surgical removal of the appendix).

"-algia" refers to pain (for example, "neuralgia" refers to pain in the nerves).

3.2.6 Words in Their Entirety

Some medical terminology are made up of a single word and do not have any prefixes or suffixes attached to them. These whole words are typically derived from Latin or Greek and are utilized in the process of describing particular medical disorders or anatomical structures. For instance, the term "sclerosis" refers to the process of hardening of organs or tissues.

3.3 Acquiring an Understanding of Medical Terminology

The sheer amount of terms involved and the emphasis placed on precision can make it appear intimidating to begin studying medical terminology. Nevertheless, there are ways that are useful for becoming proficient in medical language:

3.3.1 Separate Individual Words

When you come across a complicated medical phrase, it can be helpful to break it down into its individual pieces. Find the word's root, as well as its prefixes and suffixes. Your comprehension of these components will assist you with elucidating the meaning of the term.

3.3.2 Make some flashcards for yourself

Make some flashcards with the medical term written on one side and its meaning or a breakdown of its components written on the other side. Regularly going through these flashcards will help you improve your memory.

3.3.3 Put Your Pronunciation Into Practice

When working in healthcare environments, having correct pronunciation down pat is absolutely necessary when employing medical language. Repeating the terms out loud will help you perfect your pronunciation, and you may also look into using internet resources or mobile apps that offer such assistance.

3.3.4 Education in the Proper Context

When you learn medical terms while considering specific medical illnesses, treatments, or anatomy, you will have a much easier time understanding what the terms mean. Understanding is improved when concepts are linked to applications in the real world.

3.3.5 Make Use of Various Memory Aids

To remember difficult concepts, try using mnemonic devices or other memory aides. One way to remember the medical term "rhinorrhea" (also known as a runny nose) is to associate the word "rhino" with the nose and the word "rrhea" with the flow or discharge.

3.3.6 Investigate Available Educational Materials

Individuals interested in learning medical terminology have access to a large number of instructional resources. Consider taking a class on medical terminology, reading relevant textbooks, or studying with medical terminology-related online tutorials and tests.

3.4 Classifications Used Frequently in Medical Terminology

Categories have been established for medical terminology, with each of these categories pertaining to a different domain of healthcare. When it comes to learning and efficiently using medical vocabulary, having an understanding of these areas can be helpful. The following are some examples of common categories:

3.4.1 The Anatomy and Physiology of the Human Body

This category contains terminology that pertain to the organization and performance of various parts of the human body. For instance, "anatomy" is the study of the structure of the body, and "physiology" is the study of how the body functions.

3.4.2 Illnesses and Health Problems

These phrases are used to describe a variety of diseases and conditions that affect health. For example, "hypertension" refers to high blood pressure, and "diabetes" is a chronic disorder that affects blood sugar levels. Another example: "cardiovascular disease" refers to heart disease.

3.4.3 Procedures and Tests Used in the Diagnosis

This category contains terminology that are linked with medical tests and procedures, such as "MRI" (magnetic resonance imaging) and "biopsy" (the removal of tissue for examination), among others.

3.4.4 Medication and Treatments for the Ailments

The phrase "radiation therapy" refers to a treatment for cancer that makes use of high-energy rays. The term "antibiotic" refers to a type of drug that is used to treat bacterial infections. Other terms in medical terminology include terms relating to medications and therapies.

3.4.5 Methods Employed in Surgery

The numerous medical treatments are referred to by surgical nomenclature. The terms "appendectomy" (the surgical removal of the appendix) and "laparoscopy" (a minimally invasive surgical treatment) are two examples of these terms.

3.4.6 Subdivisions Within the Medical Field

Certain sub-disciplines of medicine each have their own lexicon of terms. The term "dermatology" refers to the study of skin illnesses and ailments, while "cardiology" refers to the study of the heart.

3.5 Regarding the Medical Terminology in the Years 2023 and 2024

The landscape of healthcare is always shifting, and the vocabulary used in medicine is always changing along with it. The following is a list of some of the ways in which medical terminology is adapting to the changing environment of healthcare:

3.5.1 Terminology Used in Telehealth

Because of the proliferation of telehealth, there is now a specific vocabulary for referring to online medical appointments. Now more than ever, phrases such as "telemedicine" and "telehealth consult" are prevalent.

3.5.2 Medical Applications of Genomics

As genomics and personalized medicine continue to make strides forward, the language used to explain genetic testing and treatments also continues to evolve. The phrases "genomic sequencing" and "pharmacogenomics" are gaining more and more usage these days.

3.5.3 Health in the Digital Age

As a result of the incorporation of digital health technology, concepts such as "mHealth" (mobile health), "wearables," and "telemonitoring" have found their way into the lexicon of the medical field.

3.5.4 Care that Is Centered on Values

Because of the transition toward value-based care, new nomenclature relating to quality metrics has emerged, such as "HEDIS" (which stands for "Healthcare Effectiveness Data and Information Set") and "P4P" (which stands for "Pay for Performance").

3.5.5 Terminology Used in Public Health

The vocabulary used in public health is always being updated, particularly in light of recent developments in global health like as the COVID-19 pandemic. The importance of phrases such as "pandemic preparedness," "contact tracing," and "herd immunity" has grown significantly in recent years.

Coding in Medical Procedures, Chapter 4

Coding in medicine is an essential part of the healthcare sector because it acts as a connection between the clinical aspect of patient care and the financial aspect of healthcare payment. This chapter looks into the realm of medical coding, investigating its significance, the coding systems that are currently in use, the function that medical coders play, and the impact of recent advancements in the field, with a particular emphasis on the state of the industry in 2023 and 2024.

4.1 The Importance of Coding in the Medical Industry

4.1.1 The Contextualization of Medical Care Services

Coding in medicine refers to the practice of turning medical treatments and processes into numerical representations known as codes. These codes are absolutely necessary for providing specific information regarding the medical status of a patient, the services the patient received, and the resources that were used for billing, statistics, and clinical decision-making.

4.1.2 Sources of Financial Gain

For healthcare organizations to be able to get adequate reimbursement for the services they deliver, accurate medical coding is the linchpin that holds everything together. It ensures that healthcare practitioners are paid properly for their services, regardless of whether the compensation comes from insurance companies, government programs, or individual consumers.

4.1.3 Obligations to Comply with Regulations

The healthcare industry is subject to a lot of regulation, and failing to comply with those regulations can result in both financial and legal repercussions.

Coders in the medical field play an essential part in ensuring that hospitals and other healthcare facilities follow the coding criteria established by the government and participate in reimbursement programs like Medicare and Medicaid.

4.1.4 Support for Clinical Decision Making

Although medical codes are most commonly connected with billing and payment, they are also extremely important for clinical decision support. Coding that is accurate contributes to the compilation of patient records that are exhaustive and accurate, which in turn assists healthcare providers in making educated decisions regarding patients' medical care.

4.2 An Introduction to the Field of Medical Coding

Coding in medicine entails giving certain alphabetic and numeric codes to diagnoses, procedures, and services rendered by a healthcare provider. These codes make it possible for providers of medical care, insurance companies, and government programs to comprehend the care that was provided to patients and to decide how much they should be reimbursed. There are primarily two different kinds of coding used in the United States:

4.2.1 Index CM ICD-10

The coding system that is utilized for diagnoses is referred to as the International Classification of Diseases, 10th Edition, Clinical Modification (ICD-10-CM). It has a huge number of codes that can be used to indicate a wide variety of illnesses, disorders, and symptoms. For instance, the number "E11.9" refers to "type 2 diabetes mellitus without complications."

4.2.2 CPT and HCPCS Abbreviations

When it comes to assigning codes to medical operations and services, the Current Procedural Terminology (CPT) and the Healthcare used Procedure Coding System (HCPCS) are the two most used options. The American Medical Association (AMA) is responsible for the development and maintenance of CPT codes, which cover a comprehensive variety of medical operations. For instance, the CPT code "99213" refers to "office or other outpatient visit for the evaluation and management of an established patient." This visit can take place in any setting other than an inpatient facility.

On the other hand, the Healthcare Common Procedure Coding System (HCPCS) provides codes for supplies, equipment, and services that are not covered by CPT codes. For instance, the HCPCS code "J3420" denotes "injection, vitamin B-12 cyanocobalamin."

4.3 The Importance of Coders in the Medical Industry

Coders in the medical field are individuals in the healthcare industry that specialize in interpreting medical information into numerical codes. Their function is complex and encompasses a wide range of responsibilities, including the following:

4.3.1 The Distribution of Code

The assignment of correct and suitable codes to diagnoses, procedures, and services rendered to patients is the primary duty of medical coders. These coders base their coding decisions on the information included inside a patient's medical record. They are required to have a strong understanding of CPT, ICD-10-CM, and HCPCS Level II codes.

4.3.2 A Look Over the Documentation

Coders in the medical industry frequently have to comb through patient files and the notes of attending physicians in order to get the information they need to assign appropriate codes. They check the material to make sure it backs up the codes that they assign, and if more information is required, they may ask the physicians for it.

4.3.3 Obligations to Comply with Regulations

Coders in the medical industry are required to maintain current knowledge of coding norms and laws. It is crucial to maintain regulatory compliance and avoid coding errors by complying with coding standards, such as those established by the Centers for Medicare & Medicaid Services (CMS).

4.3.4 The Assurance of Quality

Numerous hospitals and other medical facilities have quality assurance systems that consist in part of conducting routine audits of coded patient information. For the purpose of ensuring that their work is accurate, medical coders may choose to participate in the review and validation of either their own work or the work of their colleagues.

4.3.5 Transmission of Information

When there are questions regarding coding, medical coders frequently work together with healthcare providers and billing departments to find answers. For the sake of resolving differences and maintaining appropriate code assignment, effective communication is absolutely necessary.

4.3.6 Ongoing and Continual Learning

The medical coding industry is a dynamic one, with continuous updates and modifications being made to the criteria for coding. Coders in the medical industry are expected to participate in ongoing education and professional development in order to keep up with the most recent developments in coding standards and procedures.

4.4 Current Developments in the Field of Medical Coding

In recent years, the industry of medical coding has been subjected to substantial changes and developments, and this progression is expected to continue in the years 2023 and 2024:

4.4.1 Transition to the ICD-11

The change from ICD-10 to ICD-11 has been expected for some time now, with the expectation that ICD-11 will provide greater detail and specificity in its categorization. Coders in the medical industry need to get ready for this change, which may require them to undergo additional training and make adjustments to the new code set.

4.4.2 Coding for Remote Medical Services

The swift expansion of telemedicine has given rise to a variety of new coding issues. Coders in the medical industry need to acquire skilled in the coding used for telehealth visits in order to guarantee that these services are represented and compensated correctly.

4.4.3 Assistance Provided by Artificial Intelligence (AI)

The use of AI in medical coding is becoming increasingly common. Coding software that is powered by AI is able to review medical data, extract essential information, and recommend appropriate codes. This helps reduce the amount of work that coders have to do manually while also boosting accuracy.

4.4.4 Metrics Regarding Value-Based Healthcare and Its Provision

The move toward value-based care models establishes a connection between the amount of reimbursement received and the level of treatment actually rendered. Coding quality measurements is an important part of value-based care initiatives, and medical coders play an important role in this process.

4.4.5 Privacy and Data Protection in Cyberspace

Because medical records are increasingly being stored digitally, protecting the confidentiality and safety of patients' personal information has become an increasingly pressing concern. Coders in the medical field are required to have a solid understanding of the laws and regulations governing data protection, such as the Health Insurance Portability and Accountability Act (HIPAA).

4.4.6 An Increase in the Requirement for Coding Specialists

As more and more healthcare organizations look for experts who can assure accurate coding, regulatory compliance, and maximum reimbursement, the demand for qualified medical coders continues to climb.

4.5 The Prospects for the Field of Medical Coding

The evolution of both technology and the medical sector will likely result in the following exciting possibilities for the future of medical coding:

4.5.1 Machine Learning and AI

It is possible that AI and automation technologies will play a more significant role in the future of medical coding as they continue to progress. Coders are able to devote more of their attention to more difficult situations and quality assurance when routine coding jobs are automated.

4.5.2 Capacity for Mutual Cooperation

It is possible that more efficient coding procedures will result from improved interoperability of electronic health records (EHRs). Coders may be able to assign more accurate codes if they have improved access to the data and clinical notes associated with patients.

4.5.3 Formal Education and Professional Accreditation

It is anticipated that a complete education as well as certification in medical coding would become increasingly important. It is anticipated that the need for certified coders will be considerable, and as a result, healthcare businesses may give credentialed professionals recruiting priority.

4.5.4 Coding of the Global Health System

The demand for internationally standardized coding is becoming more pressing in tandem with the increasing globalization of the healthcare industry. It is possible that worldwide coding standards will be the result of collaborative and standardization initiatives.

4.5.5 The Practice of Specializing

Coders in the medical field have the option of specializing in a subfield within the larger healthcare industry, such as radiology or cardiology. The ability to specialize can result in increased demand as well as improved knowledge in specialized fields.

The Billing Process in Healthcare

Billing for medical services is an essential part of the healthcare business because it helps medical professionals manage their finances and ensures that they get paid for the treatment they deliver to patients. This chapter digs into the complexities of medical billing, including its relevance, the billing process, significant actors in the medical billing industry, and the influence of recent advancements, with a particular emphasis on the landscape in 2023 and 2024.

5.1 An Overview of the Significance of Medical Billing

5.1.1 The State of the Providers' Financial Position in Healthcare

Billing patients for medical services is critical to ensuring the financial health of healthcare institutions. Providers are able to cover operating costs, invest in technology and employees, and provide high-quality patient care when they have accurate invoicing and are promptly reimbursed for their services.

5.1.2 Disclosure Regarding the Patient

Patients are guaranteed transparency whenever their medical billing is correct and clear. Patients have the right to be informed about the fees associated with receiving medical care, the extent of their insurance coverage, and the amount of money that is their responsibility to pay. Trust and contentment are fostered through billing procedures that are open and honest.

5.1.3 Getting the Most Out of Your Reimbursements

There are several payers, insurance plans, and government programs, which contribute to the complexity of the landscape of healthcare reimbursement. Specialists in medical billing play an essential part in ensuring that healthcare providers get reimbursed in a manner that is accurate and reasonable for the services they deliver.

5.1.4 Compliance Requirements and Potential Legal Consequences

The observance of standards regarding billing and compliance with programs run by the government, such as Medicare and Medicaid, are of the utmost importance. It is possible for a healthcare company to incur legal repercussions, financial penalties, and reputational harm if they do not comply with the regulations.

5.2 The Process of Billing for Medical Services

The process of medical billing is a methodical and sequential sequence of processes that begins when a patient seeks medical care and concludes when the healthcare practitioner is paid for their services. An outline of the most important stages is as follows:

5.2.1 Registration of the Patient

The first step in the process is to register the patient. Collecting patient information, verifying insurance coverage, and creating a patient account in the billing system are all responsibilities of the administrative staff.

5.2.2 Documentation of the Process

The information regarding the patient's visit, such as the medical diagnosis, treatment that was offered, and procedures that were conducted, are recorded by the healthcare provider. It is absolutely necessary for there to be accurate documentation that is also exhaustive.

5.2.3 The Assigning of Codes

Medical coders are responsible for assigning proper codes to diagnoses, procedures, and services once all the necessary documentation has been completed. Because these codes express the medical services that were rendered in a format that is standardized, their use is vital for billing purposes.

5.2.4 The Generation of Claims

Claims, which are requests for payment that are delivered to insurance companies or government payers, are generated by billing specialists using the codes that have been assigned. Claims include information on the patient, facts about the provider, diagnosis and procedure codes, and the total amount that is being billed.

5.2.5 Presentation of the Claim

Claim forms can be sent to insurance companies either electronically or manually by the billing staff. It is absolutely necessary to submit in a timely manner and to be correct in order to receive rapid payment.

5.2.6 The judicial process

A procedure known as adjudication is used by insurance firms in their examination of claims. They evaluate the claim to determine whether or not it is accurate, they verify coverage, and they establish the amount that will be paid. During this procedure, there may be opportunities for bargaining and appeal.

5.2.7 The Act of Posting Payments

After the claim has been completed, the payment is distributed to the healthcare provider. The employees in charge of billing will update the patient's financial records when they have posted these payments to the patient's account.

5.2.8 The Billing of Patients

Following the posting of the patient's payment, the patient will receive a bill for their share of the overall cost of healthcare, which may include deductibles, copayments, or coinsurance. It is imperative that patients receive bills that are easy to read and understand in order to receive early payment.

5.2.9 The Next Steps

The billing staff will follow up with insurance carriers to handle any difficulties that arise from claims being refused or payments being delayed. At this stage, there is the potential for appeals as well as the resubmission of claims.

5.2.10 The Settlement of Accounts

The very last thing you need to do is check that all of the patient accounts have been addressed. Any unpaid balances or contested claims need to be resolved, and patients are counseled on how to take responsibility for their own finances.

5.3 The Most Important People in Medical Billing

The process of medical billing involves a number of different stakeholders, each of which has a unique set of tasks and responsibilities, including the following:

5.3.1 Professionals in the Healthcare Industry

It is the responsibility of healthcare providers, such as hospitals, clinics, and physician offices, to provide patients with medical care and to keep correct records of those patients' medical histories. They are reliant on medical billing in order to collect payment for the services they provide.

5.3.2 Companies That Handle Medical Billing

A significant number of healthcare providers currently contract medical billing companies to handle their billing responsibilities. These organizations help providers optimize their billing operations by specializing in coding, claim submission, and revenue cycle management.

5.3.3 Firms Specializing in Insurance

The billing procedure is heavily influenced by the activities of insurance companies. They are responsible for receiving and reviewing claims, deciding whether or not a patient is covered, and making payments to healthcare providers. Insurance providers can be private businesses or public-sector organizations like Medicare and Medicaid, for example.

5.3.4 Individual Patients

Copayments, deductibles, and coinsurance are just some of the patient financial responsibilities that come with receiving medical care. Patients are also responsible for the overall cost of their healthcare. In addition to this, they are responsible for ensuring that they have adequate insurance coverage and supplying accurate information when they register.

5.3.5 Coders in the Medical Field

Coders in the medical industry are tasked with the responsibility of interpreting clinical information into standardized codes. The correct assignment of their codes is essential to the achievement of proper billing and reimbursement.

5.3.6 Professionals Specializing in Billing

Billing specialists are in charge of managing the billing process, which includes the generation of claims, their submission, and any necessary follow-up. They verify the completeness and accuracy of the claims, which is an essential component of on-time reimbursement.

5.4 Emerging Tendencies in the Field of Medical Billing

The landscape of medical billing is continuously shifting, and major themes that will shape the business in 2023-2024 are as follows:

5.4.1 Reimbursement Is Determined Based On Value

The move toward value-based care models connects payment for medical services directly to the results and standard of treatment received by individual patients. In order to be compliant with these models, medical billing must place an emphasis on quality indicators and performance-based reimbursement.

5.4.2 Billing for Telehealth Services

The rapidly growing availability of telehealth services has resulted in the emergence of novel billing challenges. A significant priority for healthcare professionals is ensuring that virtual visits are appropriately classified and billed for their services.

5.4.3 Automation and the Use of AI

The medical billing process is becoming increasingly automated and dependent on artificial intelligence. AI has the ability to check claims for errors, discover inconsistencies, and automate regular billing processes, all of which contribute to an improvement in accuracy and efficiency.

5.4.4 Openness Regarding Pricing

Healthcare providers are required by regulations governing price transparency to make their pricing information publicly available. This pattern highlights the significance of adopting billing procedures that are straightforward and easy to comprehend.

5.4.5 Protection of Data

The digitization of medical records places an increased emphasis on the importance of both data privacy and cybersecurity. When it comes to medical billing, one of the most important things to focus on is preventing data breaches and maintaining compliance with rules such as HIPAA.

5.4.6 The Financial Responsibility of the Patient

The recent trend of increased patient financial responsibility, which includes greater deductibles and out-of-pocket payments, highlights the significance of maintaining accurate billing practices and maintaining open lines of communication with patients.

5.5 The Prospects for Medical Billing in the Future

As a result of technical improvements and developments within the sector, the future of medical billing presents a number of exciting possibilities:

5.5.1 Application of Blockchain to Billing

It may be possible for blockchain technology to improve both the safety and the openness of medical billing by making it simpler to monitor and confirm transactions while maintaining the confidentiality of patient information.

5.5.2 Real-Time Processing of Insurance Claims

The time that passes between the filing of a claim and its subsequent payment can be cut down thanks to developments in real-time claims processing, which have the potential to speed up reimbursement for healthcare providers.

5.5.3 Billing That Is Centered On The Customer

It's possible that medical billing could become more customer-centric, meaning that providers will offer patients more user-friendly billing alternatives and payment plans to boost patient satisfaction and encourage timely payment.

5.5.4 Methods of Charging That Are Easier to Understand

The potential for errors and complexity in medical billing can be reduced with the use of streamlined and standardized billing systems, which in turn improves efficiency and accuracy.

5.5.5 Application of Blockchain to Billing

It may be possible for blockchain technology to improve both the safety and the openness of medical billing by making it simpler to monitor and confirm transactions while maintaining the confidentiality of patient information.

5.5.6 Standards for Billing Around the World

It is possible that global billing standards could emerge as a result of the growing demand for standardized billing methods across international borders. These standards will make it easier for countries to engage in international healthcare transactions.

Compliance and Regulations in the Healthcare Industry, Chapter 6

Compliance with rules and regulations is of the utmost importance in the healthcare industry, which is characterized by its high level of complexity and extensive regulation. This chapter examines the crucial role that compliance plays in the healthcare business, the most important regulations, the agencies that are responsible for supervision, the repercussions of non-compliance, and the changing landscape of healthcare regulations in 2023-2024.

6.1 The Importance of Adhering to Regulations in the Healthcare Industry

6.1.1 The Protection of Patients

Patient safety should always be the primary focus of regulatory compliance in the healthcare industry. Regulations are put in place to ensure that healthcare services are delivered in a way that is safe, effective, and ethical, hence lowering the likelihood that patients may be harmed as a result.

6.1.2 The Optimal Level of Care

Regulations have an important role in both preserving and improving the quality of care provided. Regulations, which involve the establishment of standards for the provision of healthcare, promote consistent, evidence-based practices, which in turn lead to improved patient outcomes.

6.1.3 The Protection of Personal Information and Data

Data privacy and protection are of the utmost importance in this age of electronic medical records. The protection of patient data by compliance with standards such as the Health Insurance Portability and Accountability Act (HIPAA) helps to avoid both unauthorized access to the data and breaches of the data itself.

6.1.4 Integrity in Financial Matters

Regulations in the healthcare industry are absolutely necessary to preserve the sector's financial health. They make sure that billing and reimbursement are accurate, which helps cut down on fraud, waste, and abuse in the financial transactions that take place in the healthcare industry.

6.2 The Most Important Healthcare Requirements

The field of medicine is governed by a plethora of regulations, some of which have a significant influence on the provision of medical care to patients, billing practices, and overall industry operations. The following is a list of some of the most important healthcare regulations:

6.2.1 The Health Insurance Portability and Accountability Act (often referred to as HIPAA).

The Health Insurance Portability and Accountability Act of 1996, also known as HIPAA, is a federal law in the United States that ensures the confidentiality of patient medical records. It defines regulations for the use and sharing of protected health information (PHI) and requires healthcare institutions to apply measures to protect this data. These rules and requirements are intended to ensure the privacy of patients' medical records.

The Patient Protection and Affordable Care Act (ACA)

Significant reforms were made to the healthcare system by the Patient Protection and Affordable Care Act (ACA), popularly known as Obamacare.

These reforms included increasing access to healthcare, establishing insurance exchanges, and establishing standards for insurance coverage.

6.2.3 Regulations Regarding Medicare and Medicaid

Both Medicare and Medicaid are government-run healthcare programs, each of which is subject to its own distinct set of requirements. To participate in these programs and be eligible for reimbursement, healthcare providers absolutely need to demonstrate that they are in compliance with these regulations.

6.2.4 The Stark Law as well as the Anti-Kickback Statute

Both the Stark Law and the Anti-Kickback Statute are examples of federal statutes that regulate the financial relationships that can exist between medical service providers and the entities that send patients to them for treatment. They intend to combat dishonesty and inappropriate behavior in the medical field.

6.2.5 Regulations Established by the Centers for Medicare & Medicaid Services (CMS)

The Centers for Medicare & Medicaid Services (CMS) is the agency within the federal government that is in charge of administering Medicare, Medicaid, and any other federal healthcare programs. In order for healthcare providers to take part in these initiatives, they are required to comply with the regulations and recommendations that are issued by this organization.

6.2.6 Regulations Issued by the Food and Drug Administration (FDA)

The Food and Drug Administration (FDA) is responsible for ensuring that medicines, medical devices, and other types of healthcare items are safe and effective. To guarantee the well-being of their patients, manufacturers, healthcare professionals, and researchers are required to act in accordance with FDA regulations.

6.3 Organizations Responsible for Healthcare Regulation

Regulations pertaining to medical treatment are monitored and enforced by a number of different departments and bodies within the government. The following is a list of some of the most important agencies in the United States:

6.3.1 The Department of Health and Human Services (HHS) of the United States of America

The Food and Drug Administration (FDA), the Centers for Medicare and Medicaid Services (CMS), and the Office for Civil Rights (OCR), which is in charge of enforcing HIPAA, are all part of the Department of Health and Human Services (HHS), which is a federal agency that contains multiple sub-agencies responsible for various elements of healthcare regulation.

6.3.2 The Centers for Medicare & Medicaid Services (CMS) of the United States

Medicare, Medicaid, and the Children's Health Insurance Program (CHIP) are all programs that are managed by CMS. It establishes guidelines for healthcare providers who take part in these initiatives and monitors their compliance with those guidelines.

6.3.3 The Food and Drug Administration (often referred to as the FDA)

It is the duty of the Food and Drug Administration (FDA) to protect and promote public health by overseeing and supervising the quality of healthcare items, such as medicines and medical devices, with regard to their safety and effectiveness.

6.3.4 Inspector General's Office (also known as the OIG)

The Office of the Inspector General (OIG) is an independent office that operates under HHS and is charged with the mission of preventing fraud, waste, and abuse in healthcare programs such as Medicare and Medicaid. For the purpose of ensuring compliance, it carries out investigations and audits.

The Drug Enforcement Administration (DEA) is responsible for 6.3.5.

The Drug Enforcement Administration (DEA), which is a division of the United States Department of Justice, is in charge of enforcing regulations that pertain to banned substances. These regulations cover both over-the-counter medications and chemicals that have the potential to be abused.

6.4 The Repercussions of Not Being in Compliance

It is possible for healthcare organizations and individuals who are involved in the delivery of healthcare to face serious repercussions if they do not comply with the regulations governing healthcare. Some potential consequences are as follows:

6.4.1 Legal Repercussions and Monetary Consequences

If a healthcare institution is discovered to be in violation of the regulations that govern their industry, they may be subject to legal consequences such as fines and, in some instances, criminal prosecution. Persons who break the rules open themselves up to the possibility of facing legal repercussions.

6.4.2 Barring from Participation in Federal Programs

If you do not comply with the requirements, you risk being kicked out of federal healthcare programs like Medicare and Medicaid. This exclusion has the potential to have a major influence on the financial resources available to healthcare providers.

6.4.3 The Harm Done to One's Reputation

Failure to comply with regulations can be harmful to the reputations of healthcare institutions and the personnel who provide care to patients. This may cause patients and the general public to lose trust in the healthcare provider.

6.4.4 Revocation or Suspension of a License or Certification

In the event that individual healthcare providers, such as physicians and nurses, do not comply with regulations, they run the possibility of having their professional licenses and certificates revoked. This may have a significant and long-lasting effect on their professional lives.

6.4.5 Lawsuits in the Civil Court

Failure to comply with regulations may also result in the filing of civil litigation, in which patients or other parties seek compensation for injuries or losses brought on by regulatory infractions.

6.5 Emerging Patterns in Regulatory Policies for the Healthcare Industry

The regulatory landscape in the healthcare industry is always shifting, and key noteworthy themes that will shape the industry in 2023-2024 are as follows:

6.5.1 Regulations Regarding Telehealth

As a result of the rapid proliferation of telehealth services, new laws have been developed to assure the delivery of virtual healthcare in a manner that is both safe and effective.

6.5.2 Regulations for Value-Based Healthcare

Regulations are being updated to better support value-based care models, which put more of an emphasis on the results for patients and the quality of their treatment than traditional fee-for-service payment models do.

6.5.3 Standards for Operational Compatibility

Regulations governing interoperability are now being drafted in order to facilitate the sharing of electronic health records (EHRs) and other information regarding patients among the various healthcare delivery systems.

6.5.4 Openness Regarding Pricing

Patients now have greater insight into the expenses of their healthcare thanks to price transparency legislation that require healthcare providers to make their pricing information publicly available.

6.5.5 Privacy and Data Protection in Cyberspace

The ever-increasing significance of safeguarding patient information in a world dominated by digital healthcare is reflected in the increasingly strict regulations surrounding cybersecurity and the privacy of patient data.

6.5.6 Laws Governing the Privacy of Genetic Information

The development of genetic testing and genomic medicine has led to the creation of legislation that are designed to protect individuals' right to privacy and the integrity of their genetic information.

6.6 The Way Forward for Regulations in the Healthcare Industry

The future of legislation governing healthcare will be shaped by a number of rising trends and opportunities, including the following:

6.6.1 Regulations Concerning Artificial Intelligence (AI)

It is anticipated that regulatory frameworks for AI-powered diagnostic tools, treatment suggestions, and data analysis will emerge as artificial intelligence plays an increasingly important role in the healthcare industry.

6.6.2 Protecting Information and Data in Cyberspace

Regulations concerning data protection, cybersecurity, and the privacy of patient data will grow increasingly complex and stringent as the digitization of medical records continues unabated.

6.6.3 Telemedicine and Health Monitoring Done Remotely

The world of virtual healthcare is always shifting, and the regulations that govern telehealth, remote monitoring, and wearable health technologies will continue to evolve along with it.

6.6.4 International Health Regulations

It is probable that attempts to harmonize and standardize healthcare legislation across borders will become more intense as healthcare becomes more global. This will make it easier for international healthcare transactions to take place.

6.6.5 Regulations Regarding Psychological Health and Behavioral Health

The significance of services for mental health and behavioral health is propelling the development of legislation to guarantee both access to and the quality of care in these domains.

Electronic Health Records (EHR) are the topic of discussion in Chapter 7.

The digitization of patient information, the streamlining of operations within the healthcare industry, and the improvement of patient care have all been made possible by electronic health records, often known as EHRs. This chapter digs into the realm of electronic health records (EHRs), examining its relevance, benefits, challenges, major characteristics, and the growing environment of EHRs in the years 2023 and 2024.

7.1 The Importance of Keeping One's Medical Records Electronically

7.1.1 Enhancements Made to Patient Care

Electronic health records facilitate simple access for medical professionals to all of the relevant patient information, which results in improved patient care. Because of this, clinical decisions are made with more accurate information, there are fewer instances of medical errors, and care coordination is enhanced.

7.1.2 Effectiveness and Operational Capacity

Efficiency in healthcare has considerably risen as a result of the switch from paper-based records to electronic health records (EHRs). The ability to swiftly acquire patient data, automate tasks, and streamline workflows is available to providers of healthcare.

7.1.3 The Exchange of Information and Interoperability

EHRs allow for the sharing of data between various healthcare professionals and facilities, which helps to improve care coordination and reduces instances of tests and procedures being performed more than once. EHRs are able to communicate with one another without any hitches when they have interoperability.

7.1.4 Participation of the Patient

Patients have the ability to access their own health information, connect with their healthcare providers, and take an active role in their own care thanks to patient portals, which are frequently included in electronic health records (EHRs).

7.1.5 Protecting Personal Information and Private Data

Electronic health records (EHRs) come equipped with a plethora of different security measures. They protect sensitive information by providing access controls, encryption, and audit trails.

7.2 The Many Advantages of Utilizing Electronic Health Records

Electronic health records (EHRs) provide a multitude of advantages to patients, healthcare professionals, and the healthcare system as a whole.

7.2.1 Accuracy and Legibility Have Been Improved

By lowering the likelihood of mistakes brought on by illegible handwriting or misplaced paper records, electronic health records (EHRs) improve the precision and security of patient care.

7.2.2 Obtainability and Accessibility of the Resource

Because electronic records are always accessible, medical professionals can get the information they need on a patient whenever they need it, even if it's outside of normal business hours.

7.2.3 Effectiveness in Saving Time and Resources

EHRs simplify administrative responsibilities, automate processes, and cut down on the amount of time spent on manual data input, which enables medical professionals to devote more of their attention to patient care.

7.2.4 Decision Making Assistance

Electronic health records typically include clinical decision support systems, which offer alerts, reminders, and evidence-based guidelines to medical professionals in order to aid them in making decisions regarding diagnosis and treatment.

7.2.5 Reductions in Expenditures

Electronic health records have the potential to save businesses money through a reduction in administrative costs, a drop in the costs associated with paper and storage, and an improvement in the accuracy of billing and coding.

7.3 Difficulties Inherent In Using Electronic Health Records

EHRs come with a number of issues that need to be solved, despite the fact that they offer a number of benefits:

7.3.1 Expenses Incurred During Implementation

Especially for smaller healthcare practices, the initial cost of implementing an EHR can be rather high. This cost includes the cost of software, hardware, training, and the translation of patient data.

7.3.2 Instructional Methods and User Acceptance

Training is necessary for healthcare practitioners and employees in order to make successful use of electronic health record systems. It can be difficult to get users to adopt new technologies since they are resistant to change and have a steep learning curve.

7.3.3 Capacity for Cooperation

There is still much work to be done to reach the goal of interoperability between the various EHR systems and healthcare facilities. Problems with compatibility and data interchange standards can prevent the sharing of information in a seamless manner.

7.3.4 The Protection of Personal Information and Data

Because electronic health records contain potentially sensitive information about patients, concerns around data privacy and security are crucial. It is absolutely necessary to take precautions against data breaches and make certain that regulatory requirements are met.

7.3.5 The Struggle Involved in Documentation and Data Entry

Electronic health records (EHRs) can cause data input and documentation challenges for healthcare personnel, which may reduce the amount of time they spend with patients.

7.4 Principal Characteristics of Electronic Health Records

Electronic health record systems come outfitted with a variety of functions that are intended to fulfill the requirements of medical professionals and improve the quality of patient care.

7.4.1 Patient History and Demographic Information

The patient's demographic information, medical history, allergies, prescriptions, and previous treatments are all stored in an electronic health record (EHR), which provides a holistic perspective on the patient's health.

7.4.2 Notes Clinically Relevant

Documenting patient contacts, diagnosis, treatment plans, and progress can be accomplished through the creation of clinical notes by medical professionals.

7.4.3 Administration of Medications

Electronic health records (EHRs) are helpful for medication management because they include electronic prescribing, checking for drug interactions, and medication administration records.

Imaging and Diagnostic Tests, Section 7.4.4

EHRs frequently link with imaging and diagnostic tools, which enables medical professionals to access and store radiology pictures as well as test results within the EHR.

7.4.5 Requests and Prescriptions (Orders and Scripts)

It is possible for medical professionals to submit orders for tests, surgeries, and medicines directly into an electronic health record (EHR), which eliminates the need for paper orders.

7.4.6 Coordination of Medical Care

Electronic health records (EHRs) make it easier to coordinate patient treatment by enabling various healthcare practitioners to access and update patient records at the same time. This encourages teamwork among medical professionals.

7.4.7 Patient Access Points

Patients are given the ability to check their test results, connect with their healthcare providers, request appointments, and access their health records through the patient portals that are offered by many electronic health record systems.

7.5 The Changing Climate of Electronic Health Records in 2023 and 2024

The field of electronic health records (EHRs) is constantly developing in response to the shifting demands of the healthcare industry and the advances in technology:

7.5.1 Improved Capabilities of Interoperability

The efforts being put into interoperability are picking up speed, which makes it simpler for various EHR systems to talk with one another and safely share patient data.

7.5.2 Integration of Artificial Intelligence (AI) Technologies

EHRs are becoming more equipped with artificial intelligence, which helps with a variety of activities, including clinical decision support, predictive analytics, and natural language processing for unstructured data.

7.5.3 Integration of Telehealth Services

EHRs are modifying themselves to accommodate the proliferation of telehealth by incorporating telehealth platforms. This gives medical professionals the ability to conduct virtual visits and document them within the EHR.

7.5.4 Management of the Health of the Population

Electronic health records are undergoing development to enable population health management. This development will allow healthcare companies to evaluate patient data and improve the health of specific patient populations.

7.5.5 The Standardization of the Data

Efforts are currently being made to standardize health data, which would simplify the process of exchanging and utilizing patient information across the many EHR systems.

7.5.6 Health Information Generated by Patients

Electronic health records (EHRs) are beginning to incorporate patient-generated health data from wearable devices and other sources in order to provide a more comprehensive view of a patient's health.

Methods of Financial Compensation in Medical Care, Chapter 8

The process by which medical professionals and other caregivers are compensated for the care they provide is controlled by the reimbursement mechanism, which is an essential component of the healthcare system. This chapter examines the many different approaches to reimbursement, the function of payers, the influence of healthcare reform, and the changing landscape of reimbursement in 2023 and 2024.

8.1 The Importance That Reimbursement Plays in the Healthcare Industry

8.1.1 Capacity to Succeed Financially

It is absolutely necessary for healthcare professionals to be reimbursed so that they can maintain their financial stability. It guarantees that healthcare organizations are able to meet their operational expenditures, continue to provide high-quality care, and invest in their people as well as their infrastructure.

8.1.2 The Optimal Level of Care

The mode of payment for services rendered can have an effect on the level of care that is delivered. For instance, in value-based reimbursement models, the emphasis is placed on providing high-quality care in order to achieve the greatest possible reimbursement.

8.1.3 Access to the Patient

Access to healthcare services for patients is impacted by reimbursement policies. It establishes the fees that patients will be required to pay for their care as well as the range of service providers available.

8.1.4 Creativity, Inventiveness, and Technology

The manner in which medical expenses are paid for can either encourage or discourage the use of cutting-edge medical technologies and treatments, so dictating the course of future developments in healthcare.

8.2 Primary Types of Financial Compensation

Different payers, different kinds of services, and different kinds of healthcare facilities all call for different approaches to healthcare reimbursement. The following is a list of some of the primary methods of reimbursement:

8.2.1 Fee-for-Service (often referred to as FFS)

In the approach known as "fee-for-service," healthcare practitioners receive payment for each individual treatment or procedure that they carry out for their patients. This time-honored approach has the potential to motivate greater levels of caregiving.

8.2.2 Capitation [Capitol]

A capitation payment is a set amount paid for each patient for each period (such as monthly or annually). No matter what services are actually rendered to a patient, healthcare practitioners are compensated with the same amount, which covers the full scope of care.

8.2.3 Diagnosis-Related Group (DRG) (Diagnosis-Related Group)

The DRG system, which is primarily utilized in inpatient care settings, classifies patients into groups determined by the diagnoses they have received. The amount that healthcare providers get reimbursed for each DRG category has previously been established.

8.2.4 Payments Bundled Together

A single payment covers all services linked to a particular episode of care, such as a joint replacement operation, from preoperative evaluation to postoperative rehabilitation in bundled payment models. An example of such an episode of care would be replacing a joint.

8.2.5 Pay for Performance, Also Known as P4P

In the pay-for-performance concept, reimbursement is linked to both the quality of care and its outcomes. If a provider meets a certain set of performance measures, they may be eligible for a bonus or incentive.

8.2.6 Value-Based Reimbursement (also known as "VBR")

The quality of care, together with its efficiency and outcomes, are prioritized under value-based reimbursement. It frequently connects reimbursement to the outcomes of the patients being treated, which promotes high-value treatment.

8.3 The Function of Payers Within the Reimbursement Process

Payers, including insurance companies and government programs, play an important part in the process of healthcare reimbursement:

8.3.1 Personal Insurance Coverage

Private insurance firms, such as health maintenance organizations (HMOs) and preferred provider organizations (PPOs), are responsible for reimbursing healthcare providers in accordance with the provisions of the insurance plan. These provisions can take the form of capitation arrangements or fee-for-service arrangements.

8.3.2 The Medicare System

Medicare is a government program that is largely for those who are 65 years of age or older. Medicare reimburses healthcare providers using a variety of methods, such as fee-for-service, DRGs, and bundled payments.

8.3.3 Medicaid (Medicaid)

Medicaid is a program that is run jointly by the federal government and the states. Its purpose is to provide low-income persons with medical coverage. Medicaid uses a variety of compensation models, which vary from state to state, but often include fee-for-service and managed care arrangements.

8.3.4 Tricare Insurance

The United States Department of Defense runs the healthcare program known as Tricare, which serves both active-duty and retired members of the military. It reimburses providers using fee-for-service and other models in addition to the traditional model.

8.3.5 Insurance for Business Purposes

Depending on the specific plan and the contractual arrangements that have been made between insurers and healthcare providers, commercial insurance companies offer a diverse selection of payment options to its policyholders.

8.3.6 Accountable Care Organizations (often referred to as ACOs)

ACOs, or accountable care organizations, are groups of healthcare providers who work together to enhance the overall quality of service while simultaneously lowering costs. Performance-based compensation for ACOs frequently takes the form of shared savings or shared losses.

8.4 Reforms to the Healthcare System and Financial Compensation

Initiatives pertaining to healthcare reform might have a substantial impact on reimbursement procedures. Important new laws in the United States, such as the Affordable Care Act (ACA), have brought about modifications to the traditional methods of reimbursement.

8.4.1 Care that Is Centered on Values

The Affordable Care Act (ACA) and subsequent reforms to the healthcare system have encouraged the use of value-based care models, which seek to enhance the quality of care provided while simultaneously reducing costs. ACOs, or accountable care organizations, and bundled payments are both examples of these approaches.

8.4.2 Reauthorization of Medicare Access and Children's Health Insurance Programs Act (MACRA)

The Medicare reimbursement system was made more transparent with the implementation of the Quality Payment Program (QPP), which was made possible by MACRA. The Advanced Alternative Payment Models (APMs) and the Merit-Based Incentive Payment System (MIPS) are both a part of the Quality Payments Program (QPP).

8.4.3 Different Payment Models, Also Known as APMs

APMs are alternative payment models that offer novel reimbursement structures to encourage high-quality and efficient care delivery. These models have been urged to be developed and adopted as a result of healthcare reforms.

8.4.4 Financial Incentives for the Use of Electronic Health Records (EHR)

Reimbursement has been linked to electronic health record (EHR) adoption and use as a result of healthcare reforms, which have provided financial incentives for healthcare providers to adopt and meaningfully use electronic health records (EHRs).

8.4.5 Reimbursement for Use of Telehealth Services

The COVID-19 pandemic prompted changes in reimbursement procedures to support remote healthcare services. These changes were brought about as a result of the faster usage of telehealth.

8.5 Current Tendencies in Healthcare Financing and Insurance Coverage

Models and regulations for healthcare reimbursement are constantly being updated in response to developing trends and innovations in the healthcare industry.

8.5.1 Reimbursement for Use of Telehealth Services

As a direct result of the rising adoption of telehealth, reimbursement policies for telehealth have evolved to incorporate broader provisions for the covering of virtual healthcare services.

8.5.2 Openness Regarding Pricing

Patients will be able to make more educated selections as a result of regulations that place a greater emphasis on pricing transparency and require healthcare providers to make their costs publicly available to patients.

8.5.3 Factors That Are Determined By Society

In some reimbursement models, social determinants of health (SDOH) data are being incorporated because it is acknowledged that factors such as housing and food security have an effect on patient outcomes.

Data analytics and artificial intelligence are discussed in section 8.5.4.

Data analytics and artificial intelligence are being used to evaluate the quality of treatment provided as well as its efficiency. This is having an effect on reimbursement models that reward value-based care.

8.5.5 Results Reported by Individual Patients

The incorporation of patient-reported outcomes into reimbursement models is becoming increasingly common as a means of evaluating the effect that therapies have on the well-being and quality of life of patients.

8.5.6 Proposals Regarding Medicare for All

Discussions about the potential transformation of healthcare reimbursement methods on a national scale have been generated as a result of the proposals for a system in the United States known as Medicare for All.

8.6 The Prospects for Financial Compensation in the Medical Field

The development of new technologies and the implementation of various healthcare reforms are likely to have the following effects on the future of healthcare reimbursement:

8.6.1 Advanced Analytical Modeling and Predictive Techniques

It is possible for reimbursement in the healthcare industry to make use of sophisticated analytics and predictive modeling in order to establish payment rates based on outcomes and risk factors that are forecasted.

8.6.2 International Models of Payment

It is possible that global payment models will become more widespread in the future. These models would cover a patient's full continuum of care, from preventive treatments to treatment to long-term care.

8.6.3 Reimbursement Determined by Outcomes

It's possible that reimbursement models would move more and more toward outcome-based techniques, which would connect payment to the attainment of certain patient outcomes and satisfaction levels.

8.6.4 Amendments to the Regulations

Both the ongoing reforms of the healthcare system and the ongoing changes in the regulations governing the healthcare system will continue to exert an influence on reimbursement practices and to incentivise value-based care.

8.6.5 Integration of Telehealth Services

It is possible that telehealth integration into reimbursement models will continue to develop in the future, reflecting the expanding significance of virtual care in the delivery of healthcare.

8.6.6 Models of World Health 8.6.6

The establishment of international reimbursement models and standards may make it easier to conduct business in healthcare across international borders as the healthcare industry becomes increasingly globalized.

Auditing and Quality Assurance in Healthcare is Covered in Chapter 9.

Auditing and quality assurance are vital components of the healthcare sector, which ensures that healthcare services fulfill set standards of quality, safety, and compliance. Auditing and quality assurance are also essential components of the healthcare industry. This chapter investigates the significance of auditing and quality assurance, as well as their roles in the healthcare industry, important procedures, regulatory requirements, and the changing landscape in 2023-2024.

9.1 The Importance of Internal Auditing and Quality Control in the Healthcare Industry

9.1.1 Security of the Patient

Auditing and other quality control techniques are absolutely necessary to ensure patient safety. They contribute to the identification and remediation of potential hazards, errors, and adverse events that could cause harm to patients.

9.1.2 The Optimal Level of Care

The provision of medical care to patients is the focus of quality assurance processes, the goals of which are to preserve and improve care. This includes determining how effective treatments, operations, and patient outcomes are in meeting their respective goals.

9.1.3 Observance of All Regulations

In the healthcare industry, firms are required to comply with a variety of regulations and standards. Auditing helps to reduce the likelihood of incurring legal and financial fines by ensuring that compliance standards are met.

9.1.4 Integrity in Financial Matters

Auditing and quality assurance that are carried out correctly can assist in locating parts of a healthcare organization that are inefficient and wasteful. This paves the way for the business to improve its operations and cut costs.

9.2 Important Steps in the Auditing and Quality Control Procedures

Auditing and quality assurance in the healthcare industry cover a wide range of processes that are intended to evaluate, monitor, and enhance the quality of care delivery, including the following:

9.2.1 Auditing Done on the Inside

Internal auditing is the process of evaluating an organization's operations, processes, and financial systems to determine whether or not they are accurate, efficient, and in accordance with applicable regulations.

9.2.2 Auditing of Clinical Procedures

The quality of care provided to patients and their overall wellbeing is the primary emphasis of clinical auditing. Examining clinical procedures, patient records, and a clinician's adherence to clinical guidelines are all part of this process.

9.2.3 Evaluation by Peers

A procedure known as "peer review" is one in which individuals working in the medical field analyze and assess the quality and appropriateness of care delivered by their colleagues. It makes it easier to pinpoint areas that need improvement and it stimulates professional development.

9.2.4 A Review of the Utilization

Utilization review is an evaluation that determines whether or not certain medical services are acceptable and necessary, as well as whether or not they make effective use of available resources. This procedure helps keep expenditures under control while still ensuring that patients receive the care they require for their medical conditions.

9.2.5 Accreditation and Professional Certification

Accreditation and certification from respected authorities like The Joint Commission are frequently sought after by organizations in the healthcare industry. These organizations establish standards and then carry out audits to check whether or not those standards are being followed.

9.2.6 Evaluations on the Satisfaction of Patients

The purpose of patient satisfaction surveys is to collect input from patients about their experiences in the healthcare system. This feedback enables organizations to identify areas in which patient care and service could be improved.

9.3 Requirements Placed on Auditing and Quality Assurance by Regulatory Bodies

Auditing and quality control are two of the many regulatory requirements that must be satisfied by enterprises that provide healthcare services.

9.3.1 The Commission of Joint Affairs

Accrediting and certifying healthcare institutions is the objective of the Joint Commission, which is an impartial organization that operates without making a profit. Audits are carried out to evaluate a facility's level of compliance with the established quality and patient safety standards.

9.3.2 The Centers for Medicare & Medicaid Services (often referred to as CMS)

In order to participate in the Medicare and Medicaid programs, the Centers for Medicare and Medicaid Services (CMS) requires that healthcare providers achieve certain quality and safety requirements. Audits and surveys conducted by CMS are used to evaluate compliance.

The Health Insurance Portability and Accountability Act (often known as HIPAA) can be found at 9.3.3.

The Health Insurance Portability and Accountability Act (HIPAA) includes laws relating to the privacy and security of patient health information. Auditing is essential in order to ensure that data protection criteria set out by HIPAA are adhered to.

9.3.4 Health Departments in the States

Each state's Department of Health has its own set of regulations and requirements for those who offer medical care. Audits are frequently carried out to ensure that a company is complying with the regulations that are specific to a state.

9.3.5 Certification Requirements for Electronic Health Records (EHR)

The meaningful use of electronic health records (EHRs) in healthcare is regulated, and audits may be carried out to ensure that medical professionals are making effective use of authorized EHR technology.

The Office of Civil Rights (OCR) is responsible for 9.3.6.

The HIPAA standards that pertain to the privacy and security of patient health information are policed by the Office for Civil Rights (OCR), which is a division of the United States Department of Health and Human Services. Audits are carried out to determine whether or not compliance has been met.

9.4 CQI Stands for "Continuous Quality Improvement."

Continuous Quality Improvement (also known as CQI) is a fundamental principle that underpins quality assurance in healthcare. It is a methodical strategy that is driven by data to improve the quality of healthcare services and results. Involved in CQI are:

9.4.1 The Accumulation of Data

Data collection on key performance indicators (KPIs), clinical outcomes, patient satisfaction, and any other relevant metrics that need to be collected.

9.4.2 An Examination of the Data

performing an analysis on the gathered data in order to discover patterns, trends, areas that need improvement, and chances for optimization.

9.4.3 Performance Enhancement of the Process

Introducing modifications and improvements into healthcare procedures in order to address the problems that have been found and to raise the level of care provided.

9.4.4 Observation and Analysis of Results

Monitoring the effects of process improvements and assessing how effective they are in attaining intended results should be an ongoing exercise.

9.4.5 Obtaining Feedback and Engaging in Communication

Including healthcare teams in the CQI process, promoting open communication, and incorporating the feedback of all relevant stakeholders are all important steps.

9.5 Emerging Patterns in Accounting and Quality Control Auditing

In the years 2023 and 2024, the following important developments can be observed in the auditing and quality assurance sector of the healthcare industry:

9.5.1 The Evolution of Digital Technology

As a result of the increased adoption of digital tools and technology by healthcare companies, auditing and quality assurance procedures are becoming increasingly streamlined, which in turn makes data collecting and analysis more effective.

9.5.2 Telemedicine and Health Monitoring Done Remotely

The proliferation of telehealth and remote monitoring has resulted in an increased demand for quality assurance in the context of virtual care environments, which has led to the development of new procedures and standards.

9.5.3 Care that Is Centered on Values

Value-based care models put an emphasis on quality rather than quantity, which creates a demand for auditing and quality assurance procedures that center on the outcomes for patients and the effective utilization of available resources.

9.5.4 Results Reported by Individual Patients

In quality assurance, patient-reported outcomes are becoming increasingly important because they provide insights into the influence that healthcare services have on the lives of patients.

9.5.5 Artificial Intelligence (often referred to as AI)

AI is being put to use to improve auditing and quality assurance procedures by analyzing massive volumes of data to spot patterns, trends, and opportunities for enhancement.

9.5.6 Cooperation Between Computer Systems and Sharing of Information

Data sharing is being made easier as a result of efforts to promote interoperability between different healthcare systems. This, in turn, makes it much simpler to collect and analyze data for the purpose of quality control.

B.6 The Changing Face of Auditing and Quality Assurance in Today's World

The auditing and quality assurance landscape in the healthcare industry is always shifting and evolving. Possible upcoming events and developments are as follows:

9.6.1 Analytical Predictions and Models

The application of predictive analytics with the goal of identifying possible future problems and opportunities for quality improvement before they occur.

9.6.2 Artificial Intelligence and Machine Learning and Their Applications

When it comes to automating data analysis and locating trends that are relevant to quality and safety, AI and machine learning algorithms may play a larger role than previously thought.

9.6.3 Normalization and Standardization of Quality Metrics

Efforts being made within the healthcare industry to standardize quality metrics in order to improve benchmarking and comparisons.

9.6.4 Care that Is Centered on the Patient

A move toward providing care that is centered on the patient, with quality assurance initiatives concentrating on the experience, preferences, and outcomes of the patient.

9.6.5 Quality Assurance Around the World

The creation of international quality standards and audits may make it easier to receive healthcare across borders as the healthcare industry becomes increasingly globalized.

Emerging Trends in Medical Billing and Coding is the Topic of Discussion in Chapter 10.

The practice of medical billing and coding is consistently undergoing development as a result of developments in technology, modifications in applicable regulations, and variations in the nature of the healthcare environment. In this chapter, we will discuss the developing tendencies in medical billing and coding for the years 2023 and 2024, as well as the ways in which these changes are transforming the healthcare business.

10.1 The First Few Words

Billing and coding in the medical business serve as the industry's financial backbone, ensuring that healthcare professionals get reimbursed in an accurate and timely manner for the services they deliver. The translation of healthcare services into codes that are universally recognized, maintaining compliance with regulations, and improving revenue cycle management are all important responsibilities that fall within the purview of these specialists. A dynamic environment is created in the field of medical billing and coding as a result of the ever-shifting landscape of the healthcare industry, which is characterized by technological advancement, regulatory shifts, and the ever-evolving requirements of patients.

10.2 Coding and Billing for Telehealth Services

The delivery of healthcare has been profoundly altered as a result of the rapid growth of telehealth, which also has important repercussions for medical billing and coding. For the same reason that complete documentation and correct coding are required for in-person visits, healthcare practitioners conducting telehealth encounters are required to do the same for their virtual visits. These factors are driving the trend:

As a result of the expansion of coverage, precise coding is required for the filing of insurance claims. Telehealth services are increasingly covered by insurance companies, Medicare, and Medicaid.

Changes to the Regulatory Framework The regulatory bodies have revised the criteria for telehealth, including the codes for the various telehealth services. In order to maintain compliance, billing and coding specialists need to keep themselves educated.

Technology Integration: Billing and coding systems are currently being integrated with telehealth platforms, which will make it much simpler to record and code telehealth encounters.

10.3 Robotic Process Automation with Artificial Intelligence (AI)

The practice of medical billing and coding is undergoing a revolution thanks to the rise of artificial intelligence and automation. The clinical paperwork can be reviewed by AI algorithms, which can then recommend relevant codes, so enhancing both accuracy and efficiency. The following are key drivers of this trend:

Gains in Productivity Artificial intelligence (AI) and automation have the potential to drastically cut the amount of time needed for coding, allowing experts to more swiftly handle claims.

Reduced Rates of Error Machine learning models can assist in spotting errors and inconsistencies in coding, which helps to lower the chance of having a claim denied.

Adaptive Coding Systems: The most advanced software for coding is able to modify its behavior in response to alterations in the legislation and guidelines governing healthcare, which guarantees continued compliance.

Real-Time Feedback: Tools powered by AI have the potential to deliver real-time feedback to healthcare providers, assisting them in accurately documenting patient encounters right from the outset.

10.4 Value-Based Care and Reporting on Quality of Care

The reimbursement of healthcare providers is undergoing significant change as a result of the shift away from fee-for-service models toward value-based care. Professionals in medical billing and coding need to adjust their practices in order to accommodate this transition, which places a greater emphasis on the quality, efficiency, and results of care. The following are important characteristics of this trend:

Coders have an essential part to play in the process of capturing and reporting quality measures, such as patient outcomes and satisfaction, in order to fulfill the prerequisites for value-based care.

Reimbursement That Is Based on Performance: In value-based care models, reimbursement is linked to the fulfillment of particular quality and cost-effectiveness targets. This requires accurate reporting.

Coders may be asked to participate in data analysis in order to evaluate the effectiveness of healthcare providers and locate areas in which they may make improvements.

10.5 The Transparency of Prices and the Consumerist Attitude

As patients take on a more active part in the decision-making process about their own healthcare, price transparency is becoming an increasingly essential issue. Professionals in billing and coding are involved in the process of ensuring that patients have access to pricing information that is both understandable and correct. These factors are driving the trend:

The implementation of regulatory mandates has resulted in several regions' passing laws that require healthcare providers to advertise their costs for various common services.

Patient's Expectations Patients prefer to know the cost of healthcare services before obtaining care; therefore, it is necessary to have transparent billing and coding.

Patients are now expected to shoulder a greater portion of the financial burden associated with their care as a result of high-deductible health plans and higher cost-sharing provisions. This has created a pressing demand for greater price transparency.

10.6 Protection of Personal Information and Data

Medical billing and coding experts have an obligation to ensure that they are in compliance with all applicable requirements, such as the Health Insurance Portability and Accountability Act (HIPAA). This is because the protection of the confidentiality of patient health information is of the utmost importance. The following are current trends in this sector:

Enhanced Data Protection: As healthcare data becomes increasingly digital, there is a growing focus on safeguarding against data breaches and cyberattacks. This is in response to one of the most recent trends in the industry.

Challenges Presented by Interoperability Sharing data between various healthcare systems while preserving patient privacy is one of the most difficult tasks in the healthcare industry.

Data Relating to an Individual's Genetic Makeup and Personal Health The increased usage of genetic and personal health data in the healthcare industry necessitates increased security and privacy precautions.

10.7 Regulatory Amendments and the Obligation to Comply

The healthcare industry is subject to a significant amount of regulation, and the landscape of those regulations is always subject to change. Coding and billing specialists in the medical industry need to keep abreast of the newest regulatory changes because these shifts can have a substantial effect on their work. The following are important characteristics of this trend:

ICD-10 and Beyond: The switch to ICD-10 was a big change, and continual revisions to the coding system require coders to adapt in order to keep up with the changes.

Regulations Regarding Telehealth The regulations that are associated with telehealth are continually being updated, which has an effect on the coding requirements.

Modifications to Payment Models Coders are required to comprehend and apply new reimbursement structures as a result of modifications to payment models. These modifications include those brought about by the Medicare Access and CHIP Reauthorization Act (MACRA).

Compliance Audits: Compliance audits are performed on healthcare institutions, and the role that coders play in making sure that coding methods are in line with rules is quite important.

10.8 Healthcare Provision Across Borders and in Other Countries

There is a rising need for standardized international coding and billing standards to accommodate the growing globalization of the healthcare industry. This is as a result of:

Patients who travel for medical care must use a billing and coding system that is standardized and can be understood anywhere. This is known as medical tourism.

Care Provided in Collaboration Because medical professionals from different nations may work together on patient care, it is necessary for them to use the same coding and billing procedures.

Global Health Standards: Work is currently being done to unify the legislation and standards governing healthcare on a global scale. This includes efforts to standardize coding and billing procedures.

10.9 Education and Training for Working Professionals in Continuity

Those who work in medical billing and coding need to make continuous education and professional development a top priority in order to keep up with the latest developments in best practices and new trends. These are the following:

certificates: Acquiring and keeping certificates, such as Certified Professional Coder (CPC) or Certified Coding Specialist (CCS), to demonstrate your level of knowledge and ensure that you are up to date in your field.

Workshops and Seminars: Participating in coding workshops, seminars, and webinars to gain knowledge of the most recent changes in regulatory requirements, emerging trends, and coding standards.

Building a professional network in order to share information and experiences with one's contemporaries in a given sector is referred to as networking.

Maintaining Current Knowledge of Technology It is necessary for effectiveness and precision to maintain current knowledge of the most up-to-date coding and billing software and technology.

Career Advancement Opportunities and Certification in Medical Billing and Coding are Discussed in Chapter 11.

Coding and billing for medical services is a dynamic and essential part of the healthcare industry. It is of critical importance in ensuring that medical professionals receive appropriate remuneration and in keeping accurate records of patients' medical histories. In this chapter, we will discuss career development prospects and the significance of obtaining certification in medical billing and coding, both of which are vital for professionals who wish to improve their careers and maintain their competitive edge in a field that is continually advancing.

11.1 The First Things First

Revenue cycle management in the healthcare industry relies heavily on the expertise of medical billing and coding specialists. They take complicated medical procedures and diagnoses and translate them into universal codes, then they submit those codes to payers and make sure that healthcare providers are reimbursed in a timely and accurate manner. In this industry, advancing one's career is a process that entails ongoing education, the improvement of one's skills, and the acquisition of professional certificates to validate one's level of knowledge.

11.2 The Importance of Medical Billers and Coders in the Healthcare Industry

Billers and coders in the medical industry are an essential part of the overall functioning of the healthcare system. Among their responsibilities are the following:

Coding in medicine refers to the process of assigning specific codes to diagnoses and procedures based on the clinical documentation and patient records. This is necessary for the submission of claims as well as the analysis of data.

The process of compiling coded data into claims, sending those claims to insurance companies, and following up to verify that prompt reimbursement is received is known as medical billing. Billing personnel are also responsible for handling the invoices for patients.

Compliance: Ensuring that applicable healthcare rules, such as the Health Insurance Portability and Accountability Act (HIPAA) and the guidelines for Current Procedural Terminology (CPT), are adhered to in an appropriate manner.

Data management entails keeping patient records as well as healthcare databases up to date and maintaining them in order to guarantee appropriate coding and invoicing.

11.3 Possibilities for Professional Advancement and Growth

The discipline of medical billing and coding provides professionals with numerous chances for professional development and growth, which enables these individuals to flourish in their professions. The following are some examples of these opportunities:

11.3.1 Coding Specialist for Medical Records

Coding medical diagnoses and procedures is the primary emphasis of medical coding professionals. They translate complex clinical information into standardized code sets such as ICD-10-CM, CPT, and HCPCS Level II. They are accountable for making sure that the appropriate codes are chosen and maintaining current on all of the coding requirements and updates.

11.3.2 Professional in Charge of Medical Billing

Coding patients' medical information into claims, sending those claims to insurance companies, and managing the billing process are the primary responsibilities of medical billing professionals. They are also responsible for handling patient invoices, responding to concerns regarding billing, and ensuring that adequate reimbursement is obtained.

11.3.3 Certified Professional Coding (also known as CPC)

The Certified Professional Coder (CPC) certification from the American Academy of Professional Coders (AAPC) is extremely valuable and sought after. The achievement of this certification demonstrates a high level of competency in medical coding, including an understanding of the CPT, ICD-10-CM, and HCPCS Level II coding systems.

11.3.4 Certified Coding Specialist (CCS) (Coding Certification)

The American Health Information Management Association (AHIMA) is the organization that confers the Certified Coding Specialist credential. Coding in both ICD-10-CM and ICD-10-PCS is required, as this course is intended for medical coders who work in hospital settings.

11.3.5 Certified Inpatient Coder (CIC) - Certified Inpatient Coder

Inpatient coding is the primary focus of the Certified Inpatient Coder (CIC) certification, which is also provided by the AAPC. It indicates an expert level of knowledge in ICD-10-PCS coding, which is vital for those working in the healthcare coding industry.

11.3.6 A Certified Outpatient Coding (COC) Professional

The COC certification, which is provided by the AAPC, focuses on the coding needs of outpatient facilities. The CPT and HCPCS Level II coding systems are discussed in depth, making this course an absolute must for medical practitioners who work in ambulatory care settings.

11.3.7 The Certified Professional Biller (CPB) Certification Program

AAPC is the organization that provides the CPB certification, which is intended for medical billing specialists. It verifies that you have competence in the billing process, which includes the submission of claims, the posting of payments, and compliance with payer criteria.

11.3.8 Management of Health Information (also known as HIM)

Health information management experts are responsible for managing patient health records, guaranteeing the accuracy of data, and complying to compliance rules. These are only some of the broader areas of healthcare data that they work on. This industry offers opportunities for career progression that can lead to positions such as HIM manager or director.

11.3.9 Quality Assurance Auditor for Medical Coding

Auditors of medical coding are tasked with the responsibility of checking patient data that have been coded to verify accuracy and compliance. They are responsible for a significant portion of the upkeep that is required to keep healthcare organizations' financial standings in good standing.

11.3.10 Manager of the Revenue Cycle.

In healthcare businesses, positions known as "revenue cycle managers" are responsible for overseeing the entire process of generating and managing income. Billing, coding, compliance, and financial analysis are all a part of this process.

11.4 The Significance of Obtaining Certification

In the field of medical billing and coding, certification is an essential component of professional advancement. It is advantageous in a number of ways:

Validation of Expertise: Certifications are a formal certification of an individual's knowledge and skills in medical billing and coding. They provide this validation for professionals in the field. They are evidence that the person holding them is an experienced and knowledgeable specialist in the industry.

Advantage in a Competitive Market: Certifications can give individuals an advantage in today's extremely competitive employment market. Many businesses believe that certified professionals are the best candidates for open positions because they are more likely to be familiar with the standards and best practices of their respective industries.

Potential for Greater Earnings: Certified professionals typically earn higher pay than their competitors who do not hold certifications in their field. An investment in certification may result in financial benefits over a longer period of time.

Career advancement is possible through the attainment of certifications, which can lead to more advanced responsibilities and positions with a higher level of responsibility. They might also be needed for certain jobs, like "coding auditor" or "revenue cycle manager," for example.

Education That Never Stops: Numerous certification programs call for continual education and recertification, which ensures that professionals are always current with the most recent developments in their respective industries.

11.5 Bodies Responsible for Certification and Their Requirements

Certifications in medical billing and coding are made available by a number of different organizations, each of which has its own set of qualifications as well as areas of concentration. The following are two of the most well-known certification bodies:

11.5.1 AAPC stands for the American Academy of Professional Coders.

Among the many different certifications that are available from AAPC are the CPC, COC, and CPB. In order for candidates to be awarded with these certifications, they are need to demonstrate that they are knowledgeable in the areas of coding and billing. Acquiring credits in ongoing education is necessary in order to keep a certification current.

American Health Information Management Association (often known as AHIMA) 11.5.2

Certifications such as CCS and CIC are available from AHIMA. The health information management and medical coding skills included in these certifications are the primary focuses. In order for candidates to keep their credentials current, they are required to not only pass an examination but also participate in ongoing education.

11.6 Getting Ready for the Certification Exam

The process of getting ready for a certification exam in medical billing and coding requires a substantial amount of work. The following are some of the most important actions to assure your success:

Select the Appropriate Certification Do some research on the certification that best matches your professional experience and career objectives. When choosing a certification, it is important to think about both your current employment and the career you hope to have in the future.

Enroll in a Training Program: A common step for certification candidates is to enroll in one of the many training programs that are made available by colleges, professional organizations, or even online institutions. These programs offer comprehensive preparation and may include practice examinations as part of their offerings.

Review Coding rules It is important that you become familiar with the coding rules and systems that are relevant to the certification that you have chosen. This may include the CPT and HCPCS Level II codes as well as ICD-10-CM.

Practice, Practice, and More Practice: To improve your skills and increase your speed, regularly practice different coding and billing scenarios. Think about enrolling in study groups or making use of online resources to gain access to practice coding tasks and examinations.

Review the Official Content Outline for the Exam Certification organizations typically give in-depth content outlines for the examinations that they administer. Make use of these outlines as a guide for your study efforts, and you may rest assured that you will cover all of the relevant topics.

Maintaining current knowledge is essential in the rapidly evolving industry of medical billing and coding, which is characterized by constant changes in coding principles and laws. Maintain your awareness of the latest developments and shifts in the industry to ensure that you are well prepared for the test.

11.7 Keeping One's Certification Current

After obtaining a certification in medical billing and coding, it is critical to keep it current by fulfilling the criteria for continuing education and recertification at regular intervals. The majority of certification bodies demand professionals who want to be certified to:

Earn Continuing Education Units (CEUs) CEUs can be gained by attending industry conferences, workshops, or seminars; taking online courses; or participating in other continuing education opportunities. The kinds of pursuits that can count for continuing education units (CEUs) are frequently outlined in the rules that are provided by certification bodies.

To maintain certification, it is necessary for some professionals to take and pass recertification exams on a periodic basis. These exams test whether or not certified professionals have kept their knowledge and abilities up to date.

Maintain Current Knowledge of Coding Standards It is important to regularly examine and maintain current knowledge of coding standards and revisions in order to remain in compliance with industry standards.

Maintain Ethical Standards: It is imperative that certification holders uphold the ethical standards and professional code of conduct that have been set out by the certifying organization.

Maintain Your Membership: As part of the process for recertification, several certification bodies require qualified professionals to demonstrate that they have successfully maintained their membership.

11.8 Emerging Trends and Career Opportunities in Medical Billing and Coding

The field of medical billing and coding is constantly changing as a result of developments in technology, shifts in healthcare policy, and shifting priorities among patients. As you advance your career in this industry, you should take the following growing trends into consideration:

11.8.1 Coding for Telehealth Services

Coding experts need to be adept in coding virtual visits and patient encounters that take place remotely, as the use of telehealth services is expanding at an alarming rate.

11.8.2 Robotics and Artificial Intelligence Technologies

Coders are receiving an increasing amount of assistance from automation and AI in the process of analyzing clinical paperwork and assigning suitable codes. These technological changes need professionals to adapt their practices.

11.8.3 Care That Is Centered On Values

Coding and billing professionals will need to concentrate on capturing quality measurements and ensuring correct reporting as healthcare delivery models continue to transition toward value-based care.

11.8.4 Protection of Personal Information and Data

Because more and more patient records are being stored digitally, healthcare personnel have a heightened responsibility to protect the confidentiality of their patients' medical information.

11.8.5 Codes and Standards Used Internationally

It is possible that having knowledge of international coding standards may become increasingly relevant for people working in cross-border healthcare as the healthcare industry becomes more globalized.

The Future of Medical Billing and Coding is Discussed in Chapter 12

The more fundamental shifts that are taking place in the healthcare industry are inextricably connected to the developments that lie ahead for medical billing and coding. The function of medical billing and coding is always shifting because of developments in healthcare delivery, technological advances, and various payment arrangements. In this chapter, we will investigate the future of this essential function in the healthcare industry, concentrating on developing trends, the impact of technology, regulatory changes, and the role that medical billers and coders are expected to play in the future.

12.1 The First Things First

Coding and billing for medical services are crucial parts of the administration of healthcare. These experts convert intricate healthcare services into standardized codes, submit claims to payers, and make certain that providers of healthcare receive appropriate reimbursement on time. The future of medical billing and coding will be shaped by a number of important drivers of change, including the following:

The incorporation of modern technologies, like as artificial intelligence and blockchain, is redefining how billing and coding jobs are carried out. This is being driven by technological advancements.

Payment Models Are Changing The payment landscape is shifting as a result of the shift away from fee-for-service models and toward value-based care models.

A Greater Emphasis on Data Healthcare businesses are increasingly making use of data analytics and interoperability in order to improve the precision and speed with which billing and coding procedures are carried out.

Changes in Regulation The process of medical billing and coding is influenced by changes in healthcare regulations, such as the implementation of ICD-11 and continuous concerns about patients' privacy.

Patient-Centered Care The movement toward patient-centered care places a greater emphasis on the significance of correct coding and billing in order to guarantee that patients receive the appropriate care at the appropriate cost.

12.2 New Developments to Watch for in Medical Coding and Billing

The future of medical billing and coding is being influenced by a number of developing trends, including the following:

12.2.1 Machine Learning and Other Forms of Artificial Intelligence

Coding and billing procedures are becoming more and more automated and assisted by artificial intelligence. Algorithms powered by AI may examine clinical paperwork, provide suggestions for appropriate codes, and decrease errors, all of which contribute to an overall improvement in efficiency.

12.2.2 The Technology Behind Blockchain

Investigations are being conducted on the use of blockchain technology to determine whether or not it could improve the confidentiality and authenticity of medical data and billing information. It has the potential to offer a safe and tamper-proof ledger for transactions related to medical treatment.

12.2.3 Integration of Telehealth Services

As the use of telehealth services becomes more widespread, it is necessary for professionals working in coding to become familiar with the specific coding standards associated with virtual care. Coding for telehealth services is evolving into its own subfield within the larger field of medical coding.

12.2.4 Care that Is Centered on Values

Coding and billing experts will shift their attention to quality indicators and the effective use of resources as part of the transition to value-based care models, which will match payment with patient outcomes and level of satisfaction.

12.2.5 Interoperability and Data Analytical Capabilities

The processes of billing and coding are being streamlined, making it easier to collect and analyze data for quality assurance. Tools for data analytics and better interoperability between healthcare systems are driving this improvement.

12.2.6 Standards for Coding Used Around the World

It is possible that having knowledge of international coding standards may become increasingly relevant for people working in cross-border healthcare as the healthcare industry becomes more globalized.

12.3 Progresses Made in the Field of Technology

The incorporation of new technologies is one of the most important factors that will determine the course of the future of medical billing and coding. The following is a list of the ways in which technology is changing these fields:

Artificial intelligence (AI) and machine learning are discussed in this section.

Coders can receive assistance from AI and machine learning algorithms, which improves the accuracy of code assignment and suggests codes to use. These technologies also have the ability to recognize patterns and trends within clinical paperwork, which makes the process of coding more efficient.

12.3.2 Integration of Electronic Health Records (EHR) in the Healthcare System

As they advance in sophistication, electronic health record systems (EHR) will eventually be able to integrate seamlessly with software used for billing and coding. This connection helps cut down on errors, makes processes more streamlined, and improves the overall effectiveness of the administration of healthcare.

12.3.3 Block Chain Technology

The use of blockchain technology provides a decentralized and trustworthy framework for the management of medical records. It is especially helpful for medical billing and coding since it protects the confidentiality of patient records while also maintaining their integrity.

Natural Language Processing (often abbreviated as NLP)

The technique of natural language processing (NLP) can evaluate unstructured clinical notes and convert them into structured data that can be coded. It makes it easier for coders to extract information that is relevant to the task at hand.

12.3.5 Platforms for Telehealth Services

Coding and billing systems are currently being connected with telehealth platforms in order to give healthcare professionals with the ability to code and bill for virtual encounters in a seamless manner.

12.3.6 Analyses of the Data

Coders are now able to focus on capturing quality measurements for value-based care models as a result of the deployment of advanced data analytics technologies, which are being used to evaluate both the quality of care and its efficiency.

12.4 Modifying the Way Payments Are Made

A important aspect that is pushing change in medical billing and coding is the shift away from fee-for-service models of care and toward value-based care models:

12.4.1 Metrics Regarding Quality

In order to fulfill the objectives of value-based care, professionals who work in billing and coding are increasingly tasked with the responsibility of capturing and reporting quality measures such as patient outcomes and satisfaction.

12.4.2 Reimbursement Determined According to Performance

Value-based care models condition patient compensation on the accomplishment of predetermined quality and cost-effectiveness targets, placing an increased emphasis on the necessity of precise data coding and reporting.

12.4.3 Change your focus from quantity to quality

Many healthcare organizations are transitioning away from a model of treatment that is based on volume and toward one that places a higher emphasis on quality and outcomes. Coders will need to adjust to new coding rules and requirements in order to keep up with this shift.

12.5 Alterations to the Regulations

The healthcare industry is subject to a great deal of regulation, and ongoing changes in regulatory requirements have an effect on the practice of medical billing and coding:

12.5.1 The Application of the ICD-11

Coding in medical care is going to change as a result of the implementation of ICD-11, the most recent version of the International Classification of Diseases. Coders will have to acquire the necessary skills to work with this new coding system.

12.5.2 Regulations Regarding Personal Privacy

Privacy legislation, in particular those that are related to the health information of patients, are constantly being updated. Coding and billing specialists have a duty to maintain their knowledge of data privacy and security standards in order to guarantee compliance.

Health Information Exchange (often abbreviated as HIE)

The increased utilization of health information exchanges makes it easier for different healthcare systems to share patient information with one another. As a result, coders are required to monitor the correctness and confidentiality of patient information while the data is being transferred.

12.6 The Changing Role of Medical Billers and Coders in the Healthcare Industry

In response to the shifting landscape of the healthcare industry, the role of specialists who deal with medical billing and coding is evolving:

12.6.1 Working with Artificial Intelligence

Coders are working together with artificial intelligence and machine learning algorithms to improve the precision and efficiency of the coding process. While AI can be helpful in recommending codes, human programmers are still needed to verify that the codes are correct and adhere to any applicable requirements.

12.6.2 Place Your Emphasis on Quality

Coders play an increasingly important part in the collection of data to support value-based care models, including data on quality measures, patient outcomes, and patient satisfaction. This shift highlights how important precise coding is when it comes to gauging product quality.

12.6.3 Coding for Telehealth Services

The proliferation of telehealth has resulted in the development of a specific field within the realm of coding. at order to ensure that claims accurately reflect the services that were provided, coders need to become adept at coding virtual visits and patient encounters that take place remotely.

12.6.4 Considerations of an Ethical Nature

Coders are need to manage ethical problems linked to privacy and security as the usage of artificial intelligence and data analytics becomes more widespread. Coding techniques that adhere to ethical standards are absolutely necessary for preserving the faith of patients.

12.6.5 Ongoing Schooling and Training

Coders really need to participate in ongoing training and professional development in order to keep up with the constantly shifting coding requirements, technological advancements, and regulatory changes.

12.7 The Direction That International Coding Standards Will Take In The Future

The need for international coding standards and practices is increasing in conjunction with the increasing globalization of the healthcare industry.

12.7.1 Healthcare Provided Across Borders

Patients are increasingly looking to receive healthcare services from providers located in other countries, which has created a need for a uniform coding system that enables seamless billing and claims processing.

12.7.2 Exchange of Health Information Across International Boundaries

In order to simplify the transmission of health information on a global scale, efforts are currently being made to standardize coding, which is necessary to ensure that data are accurate and that systems can communicate with one another.

12.7.3 The Harmonization of Standard Operating Procedures

There is currently an effort being made by international organizations to unify coding standards and laws in order to establish a common language for the purposes of healthcare transactions and the sharing of data.

Billing for Telehealth Services, Chapter 13

In recent years, there has been a substantial rise in the use of telehealth, which refers to the provision of medical services through the utilization of technology. This expansion has resulted in a variety of changes, one of which is a shift in the manner in which healthcare services are invoiced and compensated. In this chapter, we will delve into the complexities of telehealth billing, discussing topics such as the fundamentals, regulatory considerations, coding and documentation, reimbursement models, and the prospects for telehealth billing in the future.

13.1 The First Things First

Telehealth, which is also known as telemedicine, refers to a wide variety of healthcare services that are performed remotely. Some examples of telehealth services include teletherapy, remote monitoring, and virtual doctor's visits. It has become a crucial tool in the healthcare industry, delivering a multitude of benefits to patients and providers alike, including better access to care, decreased overall healthcare expenditures, and improved patient outcomes.

Understanding the billing process is becoming increasingly important as the use of telehealth grows more widespread. Billing for telehealth services requires a specific set of concerns, including coding and documentation, as well as reimbursement methods and compliance with a variety of standards. The environment of telehealth billing is always shifting, and this chapter will provide an in-depth look at those changes.

13.2 Fundamentals of Billing for Telehealth Services

Billing for telehealth services requires many critical components that are analogous to the process of traditional billing for in-person care, and these components are as follows:

13.2.1 Eligibility Requirements and Documentation Checks

It is vital, prior to offering telehealth services, to check that patients are eligible for remote treatment and to guarantee that their insurance plans support telemedicine. Only then may telehealth services be provided. This includes contacting payers to find out whether telehealth services can be billed and whether there are any particular modifiers or conditions that must be met.

13.2.2 The Coding Process and the Documentation Process

Coding and paperwork that are accurate are absolutely necessary for the proper billing of telehealth services. While extensive documentation proves the medical necessity of the telehealth contact, accurate coding guarantees that the appropriate amount of money is billed for the services.

13.2.3 The Presentation of Claims

The charging process will start once the telehealth contact has been completed in its entirety. Claims are generated and then filed to the appropriate payer, which could be a private insurance company, Medicare, Medicaid, or even another program entirely.

13.2.4 Compensation for Expenses

It is possible for payer regulations and the particular telehealth service that is delivered to result in varying levels of reimbursement for telehealth care. When it comes to reimbursement, certain services might have a parity rate, while others might have various reimbursement schemes.

13.3 Considerations Regarding Regulations

The invoicing of telehealth services is subject to a variety of state and federal rules, each of which has the potential to influence how services are billed and reimbursed. The following are important regulatory considerations:

13.3.1 Laws Regarding Telehealth in Each State

Each state has its own laws and regulations that regulate telehealth, including requirements relating to billing and payment. These laws and regulations might vary greatly from state to state. Providers are required to be familiar with the state-specific regulations and to comply with them.

13.3.2 Obtaining Your License and Credentials

The state in which the patient resides is the one in which the supplier of telehealth services must be appropriately licensed to practice. It's possible that the requirements for credentials for telehealth services will be different from those for in-person care.

13.3.3 Equal Treatment Laws

In order to comply with parity rules, telehealth services must be compensated at a rate that is comparable to that of in-person treatments. These rules differ from state to state and can have an effect on billing and reimbursement for telehealth services.

13.3.4 Payer Policies and Procedures

Regarding the billing and reimbursement processes for telehealth services, various payers such as private insurance companies, Medicare, and Medicaid each have their own policies. In order to ensure correct billing, providers need to be aware with the guidelines set forth by payers.

13.3.5 The Ryan Haight Act (Ryan Haight Act)

With a few notable exemptions, the Ryan Haight Act places limitations on the ability of telemedicine professionals to write prescriptions for prohibited medications. When it comes to prescription pharmaceuticals, providers of telehealth services are required to comply with this federal regulation.

13.4 Coding and Documentation Within the Context of Telehealth

When it comes to invoicing for telehealth services, having accurate coding and documentation are absolutely necessary. While extensive documentation proves the medical necessity of the telehealth contact, accurate coding guarantees that the appropriate amount of money is billed for the services. Here are some important factors to take into account:

13.4.1 The Various Coding Methods

The following are some of the standard coding schemes that are usually used to code telehealth services:

CPT stands for "Current Procedural Terminology," and the codes associated with it are utilized in order to describe medical operations and services. There are codes in there that are unique to telehealth services.

Codes from the International Classification of Diseases, 10th Edition, sometimes known as ICD-10, are utilized in the process of diagnosing patients. In order to correctly identify the purpose for the telehealth visit, providers are required to use the right ICD-10 codes.

HCPCS Level II is a level of the Healthcare Common Procedure Coding System that is used to identify the supplies, equipment, and other services that are given during a telehealth interaction.

13.4.2 Modifiers for Telehealth Systems

CPT codes require the addition of modifiers in order to specify that a service was provided through the use of telehealth. GT, GQ, and 95 are all examples of common modifiers for telehealth.

13.4.3 Codes Relating to the Location of the Service

The location at which a service was performed is denoted by its place of service (POS) code. The point-of-sale (POS) code 02 is the one that is most frequently used for telehealth services. This code indicates that the service was provided over an interactive audio and visual telecommunications system.

13.4.4 The Gathering of Documents

The documentation requirements for telehealth contacts are the same as those for in-person visits. The patient's medical history, the cause for the telehealth visit, the findings of the examination, the method by which a medical decision was made, and the treatment plan should all be included in the documentation.

13.4.5 Consent Given After Being Informed

Before providing patients with telehealth services, providers ought to first seek their patients' informed consent. This consent might include information regarding the restrictions placed on telehealth, the patient's rights, and the confidentiality of the information.

13.5 Types of Reimbursement Plans

It is possible for the reimbursement of telehealth services to differ from one payer's policies and one type of service to another. In telehealth, several different reimbursement methods are typically employed, including the following:

13.5.1 Paying for the Service

Under the fee-for-service approach, healthcare practitioners submit separate invoices for each every telehealth service that they render. Providers get compensated for each eligible service they deliver, and reimbursement is decided by a fee schedule that has already been established.

13.5.2 Capitation [Capitation]

A payer will pay a fixed amount per member per month to providers that participate in a capitation model. This price is independent of the number of telehealth services that are rendered. Managed care firms frequently employ this paradigm in their operations.

13.5.3 Payments that Are Grouped Together

Bundled payments are a method of billing that involves bundling together distinct but linked telehealth services and charging for them all at once. The fact that the providers of the bundled services only get one payment for those services can result in cost savings.

13.5.4 Remuneration Based on Performance

A pay-for-performance model is one in which healthcare practitioners receive compensation depending on the quality of telemedicine services as well as the outcomes of such care. The value-based care model and quality measures are both compatible with this model.

13.5.5 Contributions to a Common Fund

Shared savings arrangements entail healthcare providers and payers dividing up the financial benefits of reduced healthcare costs brought about by the use of telehealth. The providers get a cut of the money that is saved as a result of their efforts.

13.6 Obstacles Faced When Billing for Telehealth

Billing for telehealth has its own set of particular issues, which providers need to navigate:

13.6.1 The Complicated Nature of Regulations

It can be difficult to find your way around the maze of state and federal regulations, as well as payer policies, which are all intertwined with one another. It is incumbent upon providers to maintain awareness of evolving regulatory requirements and to adjust their billing procedures accordingly.

13.6.2 Differences in the Methods of Reimbursement

It is possible for payers to offer dramatically different levels of reimbursement for telehealth services, which results in income discrepancies between providers. It is imperative for providers to have a solid understanding of payer policy and to argue for fair remuneration.

13.6.3 The Accuracy of the Coding

The use of telehealth-specific modifiers and location of service codes can make coding for telehealth significantly more difficult. However, accurate coding is very necessary for receiving the appropriate payment.

13.6.4 Documentation Regarding Telehealth

When it comes to proving that telehealth services are clinically necessary, having complete and precise documentation is absolutely necessary. It is the responsibility of the providers to ensure that the documentation satisfies the standards of all payers.

13.6.5 Consent of the Patient

It is required, both legally and ethically, that informed permission be obtained prior to providing telehealth services. In order to secure patient agreement, healthcare providers are obligated to first explain the constraints and potential dangers of telehealth.

13.7 The Prospects for Billing in the Field of Telehealth

The foreseeable future of invoicing for telehealth services presents a number of intriguing opportunities and challenging obstacles:

13.7.1 Increasing the Amount of Telehealth Services

It is very likely that telehealth will continue to develop in order to incorporate a wider variety of services. These services could include primary care, consultations with specialists, mental health services, and remote patient monitoring.

13.7.2 Equalization of the Cost of Reimbursement

Advocates are working toward achieving permanent reimbursement parity, which would guarantee that telehealth services will be compensated at the same rate as services provided in-person. Because of this, telehealth could become a paradigm that is financially sustainable for providers.

13.7.3 Capabilities for Cooperation

The billing process can be made more efficient through the use of enhanced interoperability between telehealth platforms and electronic health records (EHRs), which enables the transfer of data without any interruptions.

13.7.4 Monitoring of Patients Via Remote Connection

The monitoring of patients remotely will become an increasingly important component of telehealth. When it comes to charging for continuous monitoring of patients' health, providers will need to be able to negotiate the complications involved.

13.7.5 Ongoing Alterations to the Regulations

The billing process for telehealth services will continue to be impacted by the ever-evolving state and federal legislation, including the possibility of amendments to the Ryan Haight Act.

Management of the Revenue Cycle, which is Chapter 14

The ability of healthcare companies to practice efficient revenue cycle management (RCM) is essential to their survival. It encompasses the processes and systems that healthcare providers use to track patient income from the moment a patient plans an appointment to the moment a patient pays their bill in full. This begins with the patient scheduling an appointment and ends with the patient paying their bill. In this chapter, we will delve into the complexities of revenue cycle management, including its essential components, best practices, the role of technology, and the prospects for the future of RCM within the healthcare business.

14.1 The First Few Words

In the field of healthcare, the phrase "revenue cycle" refers to the process through which a healthcare institution produces revenue by providing services to patients and counting such services as "revenue." This cycle begins when a patient makes an appointment, and it continues all the way through the process of billing and collecting payments from the patient. It is essential for healthcare organizations to have efficient revenue cycle management in order to maintain their financial health, as this has a direct impact on cash flow, the efficiency of operations, and the overall sustainability of the organization.

14.2 Crucial Elements That Make Up Revenue Cycle Management

The management of the revenue cycle is comprised of numerous essential components, each of which plays an important part in ensuring the financial success of a healthcare organization. These components are as follows:

14.2.1 The Scheduling of Patients

The first step in the revenue cycle is booking appointments for patients. A schedule that is accurate guarantees that patients receive the proper care and that the organization is able to maximize its capacity while limiting the number of gaps in appointment times.

14.2.2 Verification of Insurance Coverage

Verification of insurance is necessary in order to establish whether or not a patient is eligible for medical care under their insurance plan. Accurate verification is helpful in determining the patient's financial responsibilities as well as the services that can be delivered to them.

14.2.3 Registration of the Patient

Information on the patient's demographics and insurance coverage is gathered during the registration process. This step is essential for ensuring correct billing and the submission of insurance claims.

14.2.4 Checking Applicants' Eligibility

Checking a patient's eligibility for particular services and ensuring that the services supplied are in line with the patient's insurance coverage are both components of the process known as "eligibility verification."

14.2.5 Coding in the Medical Field

Coding in medicine refers to the practice of turning medical treatments and processes into numerical representations known as codes. When it comes to correct billing and the submission of claims, having accurate coding is really necessary.

14.2.6 The Capture of Charge

Documenting all of the services that were provided to a patient throughout the charge capture phase helps to ensure that nothing will be forgotten during the billing process.

14.2.7 The Presentation of Claims

The practice of sending bills to insurance companies in order to be reimbursed for those expenditures is known as "claims submission." The submission of claims that are both accurate and on time is absolutely necessary in order to guarantee that the organization will be paid correctly.

14.2.8 Processing of Claims and Appeals

In the process of claims adjudication, the insurance company is responsible for assessing and processing the claims that have been submitted. The amount of reimbursement that will be received by the healthcare organization is determined through the use of this technique.

14.2.9 The Management of Refusals

Claims that are rejected or refused are handled by denial management. It is essential, in order to prevent income loss, to discover the causes of denials and make the necessary corrections.

14.2.10 Billing and Payment Procedures for Patients

The process of billing patients entails drafting and delivering bills to patients so that they can make their share of the payment. Efforts made to collect overdue balances guarantee that they be paid in full.

14.2.11 The Process of Posting Payments

The process of entering payments received from patients and insurance companies is referred to as "payment posting." This process ensures that every payment is appropriately accounted for.

14.2.12 Administration of Customer Accounts Receivable

The tracking and administration of overdue payments are the primary foci of accounts receivable management. It includes following up on patient balances and claims that have not been paid.

14.3 Exemplary Methods for the Management of the Revenue Cycle

In order to have effective revenue cycle management, it is necessary to adhere to the best practices in order to maximize the financial results and simplify the operations:

14.3.1 Instruction of Staff

It is absolutely necessary to have staff who has received the appropriate training in order to accurately register patients, assign codes, and submit claims. Continuous training ensures that employees are current with the latest developments and standards in their sector.

14.3.2 Communication That Is Crystal Clear

For the revenue cycle to run well, it is essential that departments communicate well with one another. Each department that is a part of the process is required to work together and share information.

14.3.3 The Incorporation of Technology

The implementation of cutting-edge healthcare information systems and electronic health records (also known as EHRs) helps to standardize procedures and cut down on medical mistakes. Integration with systems for billing and coding is absolutely necessary.

14.3.4 Analyses of the Data

Data analytics can be used to recognize patterns within the revenue cycle, which enables healthcare organizations to make decisions for process improvement that are driven by the data.

14.3.5 The Management of Refusals

Establishing a systematic approach to the management of denials helps identify and address common reasons for denials, which in turn reduces the amount of income that is lost.

14.3.6 Instruction of the Patient

It is possible to enhance collection rates and patient satisfaction by educating patients about their financial responsibilities and the coverage provided by their insurance policies.

14.3.7 Obligation to Conform

It is absolutely necessary to conform to the standards governing healthcare in an exacting manner, including the Health Insurance Portability and Accountability Act (HIPAA), in order to stay out of legal trouble and avoid financial penalties.

14.3.8 Ongoing Quality Assurance and Process Enhancement

The optimization of the processes that make up the revenue cycle through consistent evaluation and improvement helps to maximize both efficiency and revenue production.

14.4 The Importance of Technology in the Process of Managing Revenue Cycles

The management of the revenue cycle in modern businesses relies heavily on the use of technology. The following is a list of the various ways in which technology improves RCM:

14.4.1 Electronic Health Records, Also Known as a "EHR"

Electronic health record systems simplify the process of patient registration and information collecting, resulting in improved data accuracy and more data exchange among departments.

14.4.2 Medical Office Management and Scheduling Systems

Practice management systems provide assistance with scheduling, billing, and the submission of claims, which collectively contribute to an increase in operational efficiency.

14.4.3 Software for the Billing of Medical Services

Automating billing procedures with specialized software for medical practices helps cut down on human error and speeds up the submission of claims.

14.4.4 Instruments for Analyzing Data

The use of data analytics software helps to uncover inefficiencies in the revenue cycle and provides insights that can be acted upon to optimize the process.

14.4.5 Software for the Management of the Revenue Cycle

Devoted RCM software brings together and automates a variety of processes related to the revenue cycle, from the registration of patients through the billing and collection of payments.

14.4.6 Integrating Telehealth Into the System

The integration of telehealth platforms with RCM systems makes it possible to provide virtual care services with completely streamlined billing and payment processes.

14.4.7 Artificial Intelligence (often referred to as AI)

Artificial intelligence is utilized for the automated processing of claims and the prediction of denials, which improves efficiency and reduces revenue cycle errors.

14.4.8 Block Chain Technology

The use of blockchain technology enables safe and transparent billing and payment procedures, which in turn helps to reduce fraud and maintains the integrity of data.

14.5 The Prospects for Revenue-Cycle Management Going Forward

Ongoing technological breakthroughs and the development of new healthcare models will shape the future of revenue cycle management.

14.5.1 Machine Learning, Robotics, and Robotic Automation

In all aspects of RCM, from claims processing to denial management and predictive analytics, AI and automation are expected to play an increasingly important role.

14.5.2 Care that Is Centered on Value

RCM will place an emphasis, as the healthcare industry moves toward value-based care, on the collection of quality indicators, patient outcomes, and cost-effectiveness data for the purposes of reimbursement.

14.5.3 Billing for Telehealth Services

The growth of telehealth services will necessitate the development of telehealth billing solutions that are more comprehensive and integrated. This will ensure that claims are submitted and reimbursed accurately.

14.5.4 Use of Blockchain Technology in RCM

The implementation of blockchain technology within revenue cycle procedures will improve data quality and security while simultaneously lowering the risk of fraudulent activity.

14.5.5 Standardization of Coding Across International Boundaries

Knowledge of international coding and billing standards may become increasingly valuable for RCM workers who are involved in providing healthcare across international borders as the healthcare industry becomes more globalized.

14.5.6 Capabilities for Cooperation

Enhanced interoperability between electronic health records (EHRs) and revenue cycle management (RCM) systems would facilitate the sharing of data and improve RCM's overall efficiency.

14.5.7 Types of Payment Systems

RCM will adjust to suit these changes, which could range from bundled payments to shared savings arrangements. This evolution of healthcare payment models is expected to continue.

Management of Refusals is Covered in Chapter 15

The management of denied claims is an essential part of the revenue cycle in the healthcare industry. It is the process of determining whose claims have been denied, appealing those decisions, and cutting back on the number of times claims are denied in order to maximize revenue and preserve sound financial health. In this chapter, we will delve into the complexities of rejections management, discussing topics such as its significance, common denial reasons, the denial appeals procedure, best practices, the role that technology plays, and the future of denials management in the healthcare business.

15.1 The First Few Words

Claim denials are a typical occurrence that can have a substantial influence on the financial health of a healthcare organization due to the complex nature of the billing process in the healthcare industry. A claim for reimbursement is said to have been denied when it is rejected in whole or in part by a payer such as an insurance company, Medicare, or Medicaid. It is crucial for healthcare organizations to have efficient denials management in order to minimize revenue loss, maximize cash flow, and guarantee that patients will receive the care they require.

15.2 The Importance of Effectively Managing Rejections

It is impossible to overestimate the significance of managing denials in the healthcare industry. The following is a list of the most important reasons why efficient denials management is essential:

15.2.1 The Optimization of Revenue

A direct hit to revenue results when an application is denied. By ensuring that only legitimate claims are paid out, proper management and reduction of denials can have a considerable impact on the overall financial performance of a healthcare company.

15.2.2 Effectiveness in Business Procedures

When it comes to addressing denials and resubmitting claims, efficient denials management systems streamline administrative tasks, which in turn reduces the amount of time and resources needed to do so.

15.2.3 Treatment of Patients

It is to the interest of both patients and healthcare providers to reduce the number of claims that are denied. This guarantees that patients receive the care they require without interruptions caused by billing concerns.

15.2.4 Obligation to Conform

Maintaining compliance with industry requirements such as the Health Insurance Portability and Accountability Act (HIPAA) and the False Claims Act is made easier for healthcare firms that manage their denials in an appropriate manner.

15.2.5 Decision Making That Is Informed By Data

The data on denials can provide useful insights for the process of improving processes and optimizing revenue cycles. The analysis of patterns of denial helps discover and address the underlying reasons.

15.3 Reasons Most People Deny the Truth

The first step toward efficient denials management is developing a solid understanding of the most common grounds for denials. The following are some of the most common explanations for rejection:

15.3.1 Information That Is Either Incomplete Or Incorrect

Claims have the potential to be rejected if they contain patient information that is either erroneous or missing. This information may include demographic details, insurance information, or diagnosis codes.

15.3.2 Services Not Included in the Coverage

Claims may be rejected by payers in the event that the services rendered are either not covered by the patient's insurance policy or are not regarded to be medically essential.

15.3.3 Errors in the Coding

Errors in coding, which might include inaccurate procedure or diagnosis codes, are a major reason for claims being denied. Inaccurate coding, problems with bundling or unbundling, and outmoded codes are all potential causes of these errors.

15.3.4 Claims That Are the Same as Others

Claims that have been submitted more than once for the same service can result in the claims being denied. Errors that arise during the process of submitting claims frequently result in the filing of duplicate claims.

15.3.5 Absence of a Previously Issued Authorization

Certain services call for the payer to give their prior authorization in advance. If you do not receive this authorization, it is possible that you will be denied.

15.3.6 Punctuality of Events

Claims have to be sent in during the allotted window of time that was given by the payer. Delays in the submitting of work may result in rejection.

15.3.7 The Coordination of Benefits for Participants

Errors in the coordination of benefits can result in claims being denied for patients who have more than one insurance plan. It is absolutely necessary to correctly identify both the primary and secondary insurers.

15.3.8 Essential for One's Health

Claims may be rejected by payers if they conclude that the services rendered were not clinically necessary or did not satisfy the coverage requirements set out by the payer.

15.4 The Appeals Process for Rejections

The appeals process for denied claims is a methodical procedure that addresses denied claims and requests that the decision be reconsidered. In most cases, it entails carrying out the following steps:

15.4.1 Recognize and Evaluate the Existence of Denials

The first thing that needs to be done is to locate all of the claims that were rejected and organize them according to the reason they were rejected. Investigate the underlying reasons in order to forestall the occurrence of future denials of a similar nature.

15.4.2 The Process of Preparing an Appeal

Gather all of the essential documents to support the claim's validity, including medical records, coding information, and explanations.

15.4.3 Petition to Raise an Appeal

Please submit the appeal within the allotted amount of time and in accordance with the appeal process and criteria established by the payer. Include all of the documentation that is requested.

15.4.4 Further Instructions

Maintain constant oversight of the current standing of the appeal and maintain open lines of communication with the payer to facilitate prompt processing and resolution.

15.4.5 Resolution of the Denial

The objective is to have the refusal reversed or reprocessed in such a way that it is successful, which will result in reimbursement for the services that were done.

15.4.6 Analysis of the Root Causes

Investigate the causes of the denials and make necessary changes to the processing procedures in order to forestall the occurrence of future denials of a similar nature.

15.4.7 Instruction and Educational Opportunities

Make sure that your employees are well-versed in the payer's policies and coding guidelines by providing them with the information and training necessary to address the problems that led to the denials.

15.5 Industry Standards for the Management of Denials

An effective management of denials needs a mix of the following best practices to address and reduce the number of claims that are denied:

15.5.1 Stable and Effective Training

It is absolutely necessary to provide staff with training on coding requirements, payer regulations, and the appeals process for rejections in order to both prevent and remedy denials.

15.5.2 Automation of the Processes

Utilize technology to automate the process of claim filing, coding, and validation in order to cut down on human errors, which can result in claims being denied.

15.5.3 Appropriately Timed Follow-Up

Follow up on denials as soon as possible to ensure that the appeals process is started within the allotted amount of time given by the payer.

15.5.4 Conduct an Analysis of the Denial Trends

Conduct regular analyses of the data pertaining to denials in order to discover recurring patterns and underlying reasons, which will enable targeted process changes.

15.5.5 Communication with the Payer

Establishing open communication with payers allows you to respond to denials in a timely manner and obtain a better understanding of the requirements they have.

15.5.6 Pre-Claim Audits and Evaluations

Establish pre-claim reviews to uncover potential problems before submitting a claim, hence lowering the risk that the claim would be denied.

15.5.7 Documentation Following a Standard Format

Create standards for standardized paperwork to make certain that claims and appeals contain all of the pertinent information required for consideration.

15.5.8 Methods of Preventing Denial

The prevention of denials should be your first concern. This can be accomplished by taking preventative actions such as checking insurance coverage, obtaining previous authorizations, and conducting internal audits.

15.6 The Part Played by Technology in the Administration of Denials

Technology plays a crucial part in improving rejections management processes, including the following:

15.6.1 Electronic Health Records, Also Known as an EHR

Access to patient records is simplified by EHR systems, which in turn makes it simpler to gather the supporting documentation required for appeals.

15.6.2 Software for the Auditing of Claims

Claims scrubbing software performs an automatic examination of submitted claims for errors and inconsistencies prior to submission, with the goal of lowering the number of coding errors and claims that are denied.

15.6.3 Methods and Programs for Refusal Analysis

The patterns and trends in a company's denials can be uncovered by using software called denial analytics, which can then assist the company in identifying problem areas.

15.6.4 Submission of Claims Via Electronic Means

The procedure can be streamlined by the use of electronic claim filing, which also minimizes the probability of submission errors occurring.

15.6.5 Automatization of Workflow

The process of appealing a denial is simplified by workflow automation systems, which also ensure that all required processes are carried out correctly.

Artificial Intelligence (AI), abbreviated as 15.6.6

Through the analysis of past claims data, AI can forecast the likelihood of future denials, enabling businesses to proactively handle any problems that may arise.

15.7 The Prospects for the Administration of Denials

The continuing development of new technologies and an increased emphasis on preventative measures will shape the future of denials management.

Artificial Intelligence (AI) and Predictive Analytics

Artificial intelligence will play a more major role in forecasting and preventing denials, which will enable firms to take preventative steps to resolve possible problems.

15.7.2 Block Chain Technology

The adoption of blockchain technology has the potential to increase the safety and openness of the claims and appeals process, thereby lowering the risk of fraud and preserving the reliability of data.

15.7.3 Cooperation between Payers Made Easier

An increase in the quality of engagement with payers can lead to a reduction in the number of first denials as well as a more effective resolution of those denials.

15.7.4 Care That Is Centered On Values

The move toward value-based care models will have an effect on denials management, with a particular emphasis placed on quality measures and patient outcomes.

15.7.5 More Advanced Robotics and Automation

Automation will continue to be an essential component in the management of rejections, as well as in the optimization of operations and the reduction of human errors.

15.7.6 A Proactive Approach to the Prevention of Denial

Education, training, and continuous process improvement will play an increasingly important role as healthcare institutions shift their attention to proactive denial prevention.

Medical Coding and Billing for Specialties is Covered in Chapter 16

The processes of medical billing and coding are essential components of the revenue cycle in the healthcare industry; nevertheless, these processes range greatly amongst medical specialties. Each medical subspecialty has its own processes, codes, documentation requirements, and billing practices that are distinct from the others. In this chapter, we will examine the complexities of medical billing and coding in a variety of medical specialties. We will focus on the unique challenges and factors to take into mind in each of these areas.

16.1 Introductory Remarks

Coding and billing for medical services are very necessary in order for medical professionals to be financially compensated for their work. On the other hand, the level of difficulty of the billing and coding process might vary greatly depending on the area of medicine being treated. There are a variety of specialties, each of which has its own set of codes and documentation requirements, as well as its own set of peculiar difficulties and concerns. This chapter offers an overview of medical billing and coding in a variety of medical specialties, illuminating the distinctive traits that are associated with each area of medicine.

16.2 Care for Primary Patients

The primary care system is the cornerstone of the healthcare system and the patients' initial point of contact with medical professionals. Billing and coding in primary care encompass a wide variety of services, ranging from the management of chronic diseases to preventative care and routine checkups.

16.2.1 Standardized Codifications

Evaluation and Management (E/M) codes are frequently used in primary care settings. These codes are denoted by an abbreviation and are assigned to diagnoses and procedures related to patient evaluations and office visits.

16.2.2 The Gathering of Documents

Coding and billing in primary care need precise documentation of patient histories, physical examinations, and the processes by which medical decisions are made.

16.2.3 Obstacles There Will Be

Because they must discriminate between visits that are considered routine and those that involve complicated medical decision-making, primary care clinicians frequently face issues that are related to the specificity of coding. To back up the level of service that was provided, accurate documentation is absolutely necessary.

16.3 The Study of Children's Health

Care for infants, children, and adolescents falls under the purview of pediatric billing and coding, with a particular emphasis placed on well-child visits, vaccines, and the treatment of juvenile ailments.

16.3.1 One-of-a-Kind Codes

Along with pediatric-specific E/M codes, specialized vaccination codes are used to bill for vaccines that are administered to children in the specialty of pediatrics.

16.3.2 The Gathering of Documents

In order to ensure proper coding, providers are required to document not just the standard history and physical exam, but also the patient's growth and developmental milestones.

16.3.3 Obstacles to Overcome

The necessity of age-appropriate codes as well as comprehensive documentation can make pediatric coding a challenging endeavor. Accuracy is required for both the usage of vaccines and the administration codes associated with them.

16.4 Medicine of the Interior

Internal medicine encompasses a wide variety of medical disorders and is mostly concerned with the diagnosis and treatment of health problems that affect people.

16.4.1 Specifications and Categories

Internal medicine can encompass a variety of subspecialties, such as cardiology, endocrinology, and gastrointestinal; each of these subspecialties has its own unique set of documentation and coding needs.

16.4.2 The Documentation of Events

When it comes to internal medicine coding, having accurate documentation of thorough patient histories, physical examinations, and medical decisions is absolutely necessary.

16.4.3 Obstacles to Overcome

The extensive variety of medical illnesses, each of which may call for a unique code, is a primary contributor to the difficulty of internal medicine coding. Coders are required to have an understanding of subspecialties and the specific coding requirements for each.

16.5 Operation(s)

The term "surgical coding" refers to the process of assigning codes to a wide variety of surgical operations, ranging from straightforward, outpatient procedures to intricate, invasive hospital-based treatments.

16.5.1 Codes used in the CPT

Billing for surgical procedures is accomplished with the help of Current Procedural Terminology, or CPT, codes. Surgeons are responsible for ensuring that the codes provide an accurate representation of the surgery that was performed.

Documentation at the 16.5.2 level

When it comes to surgical coding, having detailed operating notes is absolutely vital since they supply the information that is required to support the procedure codes that are billed.

16.5.3 Obstacles There Will Be

Due to the necessity for precise coding of various surgical procedures, surgical coding is a highly specialized field that can be difficult to navigate. Coders are required to have an understanding of surgical terminology and procedures.

16.6 Radiology (Science)

Radiology is a branch of medicine that focuses on the diagnosis and treatment of various medical diseases via the utilization of imaging techniques. Coding in radiology is distinct from other medical specialties since it focuses mostly on the interpretation of pictures.

16.6.1 Codes Used in the CPT and HCPCS Systems

When billing for imaging treatments and the equipment that is utilized, radiology makes use of Healthcare Common Procedure Coding System (HCPCS) Level II codes in addition to CPT codes.

16.6.2 The Gathering of Documents

When it comes to radiology coding, having accurate documentation of the type of imaging performed, the body area that was inspected, and the findings in the report is vital.

16.6.3 Obstacles There Will Be

In order to assign correct codes, radiology coders need to have a thorough understanding of the several imaging modalities and pieces of equipment currently available.

Obstetrics & Gynecology comes in at number 16.7.

Obstetrics and gynecology, sometimes known as OB/GYN, is the medical specialty that focuses on the care of women, namely during pregnancy, childbirth, and a variety of other issues related to women's health.

Maternity Codes, Section 16.7.1

The billing for OB/GYN services typically includes maternity care, which requires the use of distinct CPT codes for antepartum and postpartum treatment, respectively.

Documentation, Section 16.7.2

It is impossible to accurately bill a patient without having detailed records of their prenatal treatment, notes from their labor and delivery, and evidence of their postpartum care.

16.7.3 Obstacles There Will Be

The necessity for codes that take into account the stages of pregnancy as well as the particulars of labor and delivery might make OB/GYN coding a difficult endeavor to undertake.

16.8 Relating to Orthopedics

Orthopedics is a branch of medicine that focuses on the musculoskeletal system and frequently involves surgical procedures like joint replacements and fracture repairs.

16.8.1 Codification of Procedures

Coding for orthopedic operations requires the use of CPT codes for a variety of procedures, including arthroscopies and orthopedic surgery.

Documentation referred to in 16.8.2

When it comes to accurately categorizing complex orthopedic surgeries, having detailed operational records and notes is absolutely necessary.

16.8.3 Obstacles to Overcome

The great variety of orthopedic treatments and the necessity of making a proper code selection depending on the particular surgery that was carried out can make orthopedic coding a complex endeavor.

16.9 Relating to Dermatology

The diagnosis and treatment of various skin problems and diseases are the primary focuses of dermatology.

16.9.1 Codes for the Removal of Lesions

When it comes to coding dermatology, it is common practice to include codes for the excision of skin lesions like moles and warts.

16.9.2 Details of the Documentation

Coding in dermatology relies heavily on detailed and precise descriptions of skin lesions, which must include information on the lesion's size, location, and removal procedure.

16.9.3 Obstacles There Will Be

Coders in the field of dermatology need to be familiar with a wide variety of skin disorders as well as the proper codes for lesion removal.

16.10 Eye and Vision Care

The diagnosis and treatment of various eye illnesses and ailments are the primary objectives of ophthalmology.

16.10.1 Codes for Eye Examinations

Coding in ophthalmology encompasses not only codes for thorough eye exams but also codes for operations such as cataract surgery and codes for the prescription of eyeglasses.

16.10.2 Documentation (Documentation)

It is absolutely necessary for correct ophthalmology coding to have comprehensive documentation of the findings of the eye exam, diagnostic testing, and surgical reports.

16.10.3 Obstacles There Will Be

Coding in ophthalmology needs expertise with the various kinds of eye exams, diagnostic tests, and procedures, each of which has its own distinct code set.

16.11 Conditions Relating to the Mind and the Behavioral Health

Services related to mental health and behavioral health include evaluation and treatment of psychological and emotional illnesses.

16.11.1 Codes of Practice for Evaluation and Management

E/M codes are frequently utilized by psychiatrists and psychologists for the purpose of billing for office visits and examinations.

16.11.2 Codes Relating to Behavioral Health

Codes specific to behavioral health services can be found in the CPT manual; examples include those for psychotherapy and psychological testing.

16.11.3 Documentation (Documentation)

When it comes to mental and behavioral health coding, having comprehensive documentation of patient assessments, treatment plans, and therapy sessions is absolutely necessary.

16.11.4 Obstacles There Will Be

Coding for mental health can be difficult since it requires an accurate representation of the patient's emotional and psychological condition to be entered. Coders are required to have a comprehensive understanding of the complexities of mental health diagnosis and therapy.

16.12 The use of anesthesia

The process of administering anaesthetic in preparation for and during medical and surgical procedures is known as "anesthesia coding."

16.12.1 Codes Relating to Anesthetics

When billing for anesthesia services, certain CPT codes are used, which take into account a number of variables, including the patient's age, current health status, and the degree of difficulty of the surgery.

16.12.2 Documentation (Documentation)

The sort of anesthetic that was given to the patient, their reaction to it, and any difficulties must all be documented by the anesthesia provider.

16.12.3 Obstacles There Will Be

Coding for anesthesia can be difficult because it requires selecting the correct code according to the procedure being performed and the condition of the patient.

16.13 Acute Care and Disaster Medicine

The diagnosis and treatment of acute diseases that pose a risk to the patient's life are the primary focuses of emergency medicine, which is practiced in hospital emergency rooms.

E/M Codes, Section 16.13.1

E/M codes are frequently utilized in emergency medicine for the purpose of billing for the examination and management of patients in the emergency department.

16.13.2 Codes of Operative Procedure

Emergency medicine may also involve procedure codes for treatments such as wound repairs or fracture reductions, in addition to E/M codes.

16.13.3 Documentation (Documentation)

It is absolutely necessary for correct invoicing to have detailed record of the patient's health, history, and the services that were performed.

16.13.4 Obstacles There Will Be

Due to the time-sensitive nature of emergency care, coding for emergency medicine can be frenetic and difficult. Coders are tasked with providing an accurate representation of the degree of service extended during emergency situations.

16.14 The Study of Cancer

The diagnosis and treatment of cancer are the purview of oncology, which include such modalities as chemotherapy, radiation therapy, and surgical operations.

Chemotherapy Codes, Section 16.14.1

Billing for oncology services must include particular codes to account for chemotherapy and infusion services.

Codes for Radiation Therapy in Section 16.14.2

The CPT codes that are used to bill for radiation therapy treatments correspond to the nature and degree of difficulty of the treatment being provided.

Documentation at the 16.14.3 level

When it comes to oncology coding, having accurate documentation of chemotherapy medicines, doses, and administration, in addition to facts regarding radiation therapy, is essential.

16.14.4 Obstacles There Will Be

The wide variety of chemotherapy medications and treatment plans, in addition to the requirement to precisely record radiation therapy particulars, can make oncology coding a difficult endeavor to undertake.

Physical therapy and rehabilitation come in at number 16.15.

Patients often require assistance recovering from injuries or procedures in order to restore their mobility. Physical therapy and rehabilitation can provide this assistance.

16.15.1 Codes of the CPT

CPT codes are used in the billing process for services related to physical therapy and rehabilitation. These codes indicate therapeutic exercises, manual therapy, and modalities.

Documentation at the 16.15.2 level

Coding and billing require extensive documenting of the patient's condition, treatment plan, and progress. This paperwork should be as detailed as possible.

16.15.3 Obstacles to Overcome

Coding for physical therapy and rehabilitation requires knowledge of the individual services that are rendered and the codes that are assigned to those services.

16.16 Geriatrics and Old Age

Geriatrics is the area of medicine that focuses on the treatment of elderly patients and the management of health problems that are associated with aging.

16.16.1 Codes for the Assessment of Geriatric Patients

When it comes to drug management, care coordination, and complete geriatric assessments, geriatric medicine may require its own unique set of billing codes.

Documentation at the 16.16.2 level

When it comes to geriatric coding, having thorough documentation of the patient's medical history, functional status, and cognitive evaluations is absolutely necessary.

16.16.3 Obstacles There Will Be

Coders must appropriately document the patient's condition and care plan in order to perform geriatric coding. Geriatric coding may require the assessment of complex health conditions connected to aging.

16.17 Urology Urology

Urology is the medical specialty that deals with the diagnosis and treatment of disorders that affect the male reproductive organs and the urinary system.

Procedure Codes, Section 16.17.1

CPT codes for urological procedures such cystoscopies, lithotripsies, and urodynamic testing are included in the field of urology coding.

Documentation at the 16.17.2 level

Urology coding requires precise recording of the procedure that was carried out, the findings, and any difficulties that arose as a result.

16.17.3 Obstacles There Will Be

Urology coding can be difficult since it requires selecting the proper code based on the particular operation and findings of each patient.

16.18 Immunology and Allergic Diseases

The diagnosis and treatment of conditions such as asthma, allergies, and diseases of the immune system are the primary focuses of allergy and immunology.

16.18.1 Codes for Allergic Reaction Testing

The coding used in allergy and immunology encompasses allergy testing, treatment, and office visits, among other things.

Documentation referred to in 16.18.2

Coding requires extensive, well-documented information regarding the outcomes of allergy testing, the delivery of immunotherapy, and patient evaluations.

16.18.3 Obstacles There Will Be

When it comes to coding for allergy and immunology, you need to be familiar with the various kinds of allergy testing as well as the relevant codes for each.

16.19 The Anatomic and Surgical Pathology

The diagnosis of diseases and disorders sometimes requires an anatomic pathologist to investigate organs, tissues, and even individual cells.

16.19.1 Codes Used in Pathology

CPT codes are utilized in anatomic pathology coding for services such as tissue exams, cytology, and pathology consultations.

16.19.2 Documentation (Documentation)

When it comes to anatomic pathology coding, having accurate documentation of the specimen, the examination, and the findings is quite necessary.

16.19.3 Obstacles There Will Be

Coding in anatomic pathology can be difficult due to the wide range of specimens and examinations that must be performed, as well as the necessity of making precise code selections.

16.20 Chiropractic Care and Adjustments

Adjustments to the patient's spine are a common part of chiropractic treatment, which focuses on the diagnosis and treatment of musculoskeletal disorders.

CPT Codes as of 16.20.1

Billing for chiropractic services, including spinal manipulative therapy and other chiropractic services, is accomplished with specialized CPT codes.

Documentation regarding 16.20.2

When it comes to chiropractic coding, having detailed documentation of the patient's condition, treatment plan, and the particular manipulations that were performed is absolutely necessary.

16.20.3 Obstacles to Overcome

Coding for chiropractic care needs precise recording of the number of manipulations performed, the type of manipulations used, and the necessity of those treatments.

16.21 Coding and Billing Requirements for Special Procedures

Some fields of expertise involve one-of-a-kind processes and services, which in turn call for distinct forms of documentation and coding:

Medicine for Sleeping at 16.21.1

Polysomnography, home sleep apnea testing, and the treatment of sleep disorders utilizing specialized codes and documentation are all examples of what can be included in sleep medicine.

16.21.2 Treatment and Management of Pain

Interventional pain procedures and the use of drugs to treat chronic pain are common components of pain management. Both of these components, which require specific codes and documentation, fall under the umbrella of "pain management."

16.21.3 Complementary and Alternative Medicine

Acupuncture and chiropractic therapy are two examples of the types of treatment that fall under the umbrella of integrative and complementary medicine. Each of these modalities has its own set of coding and documentation requirements.

Nuclear medicine comes in at 16.21.4.

Nuclear medicine encompasses imaging for diagnostic purposes as well as therapies that make use of radioactive materials; as a result, particular codes and paperwork are required.

16.22 Coding and Billing for Telemedicine Services

Because of its growing significance in the healthcare industry, telemedicine necessitates the adoption of particular billing and coding procedures:

16.22.1 Services of a Telehealth Nature

Virtual patient visits, remote patient monitoring, and other telehealth services are all covered by the telehealth codes.

Documentation as of 16.22.2

Coding for telemedicine requires extensive documentation, which should include information on the location of the patient, the location of the provider, and the services that were rendered.

16.22.3 Obstacles There Will Be

Because of the requirement to comply with state and federal standards, as well as licensure and billing guidelines, telemedicine coding can be a challenging endeavor.

Legal and Ethical Considerations in Medical Billing and Coding is the Topic of Chapter 17

In the field of medicine, medical billing and coding are not only necessary for effective revenue cycle management, but they are also subject to a convoluted web of legal and ethical considerations. In other words, they are a double-edged sword. A few of the most important factors that must be adhered to with utmost precision are the accuracy of the codes, the protection of the patient's personal information, and the observance of the regulations. In this chapter, we will delve into the legal and ethical aspects of medical billing and coding. Specifically, we will investigate the most important laws and regulations, ethical norms, and the impact that these factors have on the healthcare business.

17.1 The First Few Words

The process of translating medical services into codes that are used by insurers to determine reimbursement is known as medical billing and coding. This process serves as the financial backbone of the healthcare business. Accuracy and honesty throughout this process are absolutely necessary in order to guarantee that those who offer medical treatment will be fairly compensated for their efforts. However, this approach does not come without its fair share of ethical and legal complications. This chapter will provide light on the rules, regulations, and principles that govern this area by examining the legal and ethical aspects that are involved in medical billing and coding.

17.2 The Existing Legal Structure

The legal framework that encompasses medical billing and coding is complex, consisting of a variety of rules and regulations at the federal and state levels. These were enacted with the goal of ensuring that the reimbursement process is accurate and equitable. It is absolutely necessary for healthcare organizations and professionals involved in billing and coding to comprehend these regulatory obligations and act in accordance with them.

HIPAA stands for the Health Insurance Portability and Accountability Act.

Protecting patients' protected health information (PHI) is the primary objective of the Health Insurance Portability and Accountability Act, most generally referred to as HIPAA. This law was passed by the federal government in 1996. Even though it is not directly connected to medical coding and billing, it plays an extremely important part in protecting the confidentiality and safety of patient information across the whole healthcare system. When dealing with patient information, healthcare practitioners and billing professionals are required to comply with the severe regulations outlined in HIPAA.

17.2.2 The Federal Fraud and Claims Act

The federal False Claims Act (FCA) is a statute that makes individuals and organizations liable for their actions if they commit fraud against government programs. It is important to remember that the Fair Credit Billing Act (FCA) targets the submission of incorrect or fraudulent claims to federal healthcare programs like Medicare and Medicaid. This makes the FCA relevant in the context of medical billing and coding. Fines and other penalties of a significant nature may be imposed for infractions of the FCA.

17.2.3 Anti-Kickback Statute of the United States

According to the Anti-Kickback Statute, it is illegal for healthcare professionals to offer, pay, solicit, or receive money in exchange for the creation of business involving any federal healthcare program. Additionally, it is illegal for healthcare providers to offer remuneration in exchange for patient referrals. This law is absolutely necessary for eliminating dishonest billing practices and preserving the honesty of the healthcare services that are provided.

17.2.4 Statute of Stark

The Stark Law, which is often referred to by its formal name, the Physician Self-Referral Law, places limitations on the ability of physicians to recommend patients for certain defined medical services to organizations with whom they have financial links. Compliance with the Stark Law is absolutely necessary for the elimination of any conflicts of interest, any of which could result in unethical billing procedures.

17.2.5 Health Care Affordability Act of 2010

The Patient Protection and Affordable Care Act (ACA) includes features such as reforms to the private health insurance market, the development of health insurance exchanges, and enhanced coverage for preventive treatments that have the potential to effect medical billing and coding. For correct billing and reimbursement, compliance with the regulations of the ACA is absolutely necessary.

17.2.6 The Regulations of the State

In addition to being governed by federal statutes, medical billing and coding must also comply with standards that are unique to each state. It is possible for states to have their own requirements for billing and coding, restrictions regarding the license of professionals, and insurance legislation that effect the process of payment. Legal considerations at both the federal and state levels must be navigated by organizations in the healthcare industry.

17.3 Ethical Principles and Requirements

Ethical considerations in medical billing and coding are equally significant since they protect the patients' welfare and are the foundation upon which trust in the healthcare system is built. Guidelines for ethics act as a compass for professionals working in this industry, assisting them in making judgments that are morally correct and maintaining the greatest standards of integrity possible.

17.3.1 Standards of Ethical Conduct for Members of the American Health Information Management Association (AHIMA)

The American Health Information Management Association (AHIMA) Code of Ethics offers a comprehensive framework for professionals working in healthcare information management, including medical coders. It places a strong emphasis on values such as honesty, discretion, and ongoing education and training for professionals. It is absolutely essential to adhere to this code in order to protect the confidentiality of patient information and to guarantee ethical behavior among those working in this industry.

17.3.2 The Code of Ethics Adopted by the American Academy of Professional Coders (AAPC)

The American Academy of Professional Coders (AAPC), which is a premier organization for medical coding experts, has its very own Code of Ethics, which encourages professionalism, integrity, and respect for patient confidentiality. It is absolutely necessary for individuals who are certified coders as well as those who are seeking certification to abide by the AAPC Code of Ethics.

17.3.3 Ethical Standards Established by the National Association for Healthcare Revenue Integrity (NAHRI)

The NAHRI Code of Ethics stresses the necessity of being truthful, accurate, and compliant when it comes to maintaining revenue integrity and providing compliant healthcare. Professionals in the various aspects of revenue cycle management, such as billing and coding, can look to this code for direction.

17.3.4 Ethical Challenges Facing Those Who Work in Medical Billing and Coding

Coders and billers in the medical industry may run into uncomfortable moral conundrums in the course of their profession. Concerns regarding upcoding (the practice of assigning codes that represent more complexity or cost than the services given), unbundling (the practice of individually invoicing components of a procedure that should be invoiced together), and fraudulent billing are examples of some of the potential issues that may arise as a result of this practice. Dealing with these conundrums calls for moral discernment as well as a dedication to upholding the greatest professional standards.

17.4 The Effects of Being in Compliance with Laws and Codes of Ethics

In the field of medical billing and coding, the significance of adhering to all applicable laws and standards of ethical conduct cannot be emphasized. Failure to comply with regulations can have devastating effects, not just on individual practitioners but also on healthcare institutions. It is essential to have a solid understanding of the implications of either adhering to or violating legal and ethical standards.

17.4.1 Damage to One's Reputation

The reputation of healthcare professionals and organizations might be damaged if they do not adhere to the legal and ethical standards that are in place. Allegations of false billing or breaches of patients' privacy can damage patients' trust and have effects that linger for a long time.

17.4.2 Repercussions From the Law

Infractions of state and federal laws, such as the False Claims Act or the Health Insurance Portability and Accountability Act (HIPAA), can result in civil and criminal consequences, including monetary fines, jail time, and disqualification from participation in government healthcare programs.

17.4.3 The Cost to the Organization

Failure to comply with standards governing billing and coding can result in the loss of revenue as a result of denied claims, the need to pay legal fees and fines, and the requirement to conduct expensive audits and investigations.

17.4.4 Damage to the Patient

improper coding or billing methods have the potential to cause patients to suffer harm if they lead to improper treatments, delays in care, or the unlawful use of protected health information.

17.4.5 Repercussions for One's Profession

If a professional in the medical billing and coding industry engages in activities that violate professional ethics or the law, they may be subject to disciplinary action, which may include the loss of their certification and their professional reputation.

17.5 Conformity Assessment and Programs

It is common practice for healthcare businesses to develop compliance procedures in order to successfully traverse the complicated environment of legal and ethical considerations in medical billing and coding. These programs are intended to ensure that the organization as a whole as well as its workers comply with all applicable laws, regulations, and ethical standards.

17.5.1 Components that Complying Programs Should Have

The following components are commonly seen in effective compliance programs:

17.5.1.1 Policies and Procedures That Are Composed In Writing

Policies and procedures that are both clear and comprehensive, outlining the firm's commitment to legal and ethical compliance, are desirable in any organization.

17.5.1.2 Officer Designated to Oversee Compliance

The designation of a compliance officer as the individual in charge of monitoring the program and resolving any problems related to compliance.

17.5.1.3 The Education and Training of Staff Members

Training programs for employees that educate them on legal and ethical norms, ensuring that they comprehend the obligations that are assigned to them.

Auditing and Watching Over Everything 17.5.1.4

Audits and monitoring of the billing and coding procedures on a regular basis in order to detect and address any compliance concerns that arise.

17.5.1.5 Systematized Methods of Reporting

Employees should be able to report possible compliance issues without fear of retaliation using the mechanisms provided.

17.5.1.6 Course of Action to Be Taken

A procedure for dealing with violations of compliance, which may involve remedial action, restitution, and modifications to policies and procedures to prevent similar violations in the future.

17.5.2 Constant and Continued Vigilance

In order to remain in compliance with ever-evolving rules, regulations, and ethical standards, compliance programs demand constant vigilance. It is imperative that businesses working in healthcare keep abreast of the latest legal and ethical advancements in the industry and adapt their programs accordingly.

17.6 Studies of Specific Cases

Let's take a look at two case studies that illustrate the practical implications of legal and ethical issues in medical billing and coding. These case studies highlight the potential consequences of non-compliance and the need of adhering to established standards. The purpose of this exercise is to illustrate the practical implications of legal and ethical considerations in medical billing and coding.

17.6.1 An Example of Upcoding as a Case Study 1

A medical coder who works for a major healthcare institution may find themselves under pressure from their supervisor to assign higher-level codes for patient visits, even if the services given may not fulfill the criteria for the higher code. In order to prevent any potential conflicts, the coder complies with the supervisor's request, although they are afterwards scrutinized for upcoding. The coder may face legal action, monetary fines, and harm to their professional reputation as a result of the consequences.

17.6.2 The Case Study 2: An Invasion of Privacy

A billing expert at a modest medical practice sends an email with a patient's billing statement to the incorrect recipient, so making the patient's personal as well as medical information publicly available. The breach constitutes a violation of the privacy standards established by HIPAA, which leads to an inquiry by the Office for Civil Rights (OCR) and the possibility of penalties, in addition to reputational harm to the practice.

Updates to the International Classification of Diseases (ICD) is the topic of discussion in Chapter 18.

The International Classification of Diseases, or ICD for short, is a system that is acknowledged all over the world for classifying and coding diseases, disorders, and a variety of other health-related issues. The International Classification of Diseases (ICD) is a vital resource in the healthcare industry and plays an important role in medical billing, public health, and clinical research. It is managed by the World Health Organization (WHO). This chapter examines the significance of the International Classification of Diseases (ICD) system, its history, and the most recent changes to ICD-11, putting light on its function in contemporary healthcare.

18.1 The First Few Words

The International Classification of Diseases, also known as the ICD, is a method that is utilized for the purpose of categorizing illnesses and other disorders that are associated with one's state of health on a global scale. The International Classification of Diseases (ICD) is a key component in healthcare, epidemiology, health management, and medical billing. The World Health Organization (WHO) is responsible for developing and maintaining the ICD. This chapter examines the relevance of the ICD system, its historical development, as well as the most recent improvements that were implemented in ICD-11.

18.2 The Importance of Using the ICD

The International Classification of Diseases (ICD) performs a number of essential roles in the medical and public health arenas, including the following:

18.2.1 Establishing a Common Standard for Disease Classification

The International Classification of Diseases (ICD) provides a framework that is standardized and uniform for classifying and coding diseases and health problems. This ensures that medical practitioners all around the world utilize the same language.

18.2.2 Making the Data Collection Process Easier

The International Classification of Diseases (ICD) is used by healthcare systems, public health authorities, and researchers to gather and analyze data pertaining to health. These data are extremely helpful for monitoring the prevalence of disease, determining trends, and making preparations for healthcare services.

18.2.3 Providing Assistance with Medical Billing and Reimbursement

The ICD system is essential to both the billing process for medical services and the filing of insurance claims. The correct use of ICD coding enables medical professionals to communicate with patients' insurance regarding the nature of a patient's ailment, which in turn enables accurate reimbursement for services given.

18.2.4 Improving Patient Care and Clinical Services

The International Classification of Diseases (ICD) is a system that helps medical professionals diagnose and treat patients by providing standardized terminology and codes for various medical diseases. This facilitates straightforward communication and cuts down on the number of errors.

18.2.5 Having an Effect on the Policy Regarding Public Health

The data from the ICD are used to inform the policies and interventions in public health. It helps to identify disease outbreaks, track health trends, and provide direction for preventative efforts.

18.3 A Brief Overview of the ICD's Past

ICD development has a long and illustrious history, and it has progressed throughout the years to adapt to the ever-evolving requirements of the medical community:

18.3.1 Earlier Systematizations of Classification

The International Classification of Diseases (ICD) can be traced back to the 18th and 19th centuries, when early attempts were made to categorize diseases and causes of death. These early efforts laid the groundwork for the ICD system. These systems were simplistic and did not have the reach that the ICD does across the globe.

18.3.2 The Establishment of the ICD

Late in the 19th century, under the direction of the International Statistical Institute, the International Classification of Diseases (ICD) was formally formed. In 1893, the first version of what would later become known as the Bertillon Classification was released.

18.3.3 Developing New Material and Making Changes

As the International Classification of Diseases (ICD) expanded over the course of numerous editions, it grew to incorporate a wider variety of diseases and health problems. The publication of the ICD-10 in 1992 marked a significant milestone since it offered categories and coding that were more specific.

18.3.4 The Development of the ICD-11

The most recent version of the system, known as ICD-11, was created over the course of a decade and was made available by the WHO in June of 2018. It reflects developments in medical knowledge, changes in the landscape of healthcare, as well as the need for improved disease classification.

18.4 Recent Changes to the ICD-11

When compared to its predecessor, ICD-10, the International Classification of Diseases, Eleventh Revision (ICD-11) marks a significant advancement in disease classification, incorporating a large number of changes and enhancements, including the following:

18.4.1 Format in a Structured Manner

The ICD-11 uses a format that is both structured and user-friendly, which makes it easier to use and results in more accurate classification. It features an intuitive user interface and better capability for doing searches.

18.4.2 Terms with Improved Accuracy

The vocabulary in ICD-11 has been changed to fit more closely with modern medical practice, which allows it to accommodate the changes and advancements that have taken place in the area. It offers definitions and explanations of diseases and ailments that have been brought up to date.

18.4.3 The Implementation of New Conditions

ICD-11 includes diseases and conditions that did not exist in ICD-10, reflecting the changing landscape of health challenges such as new infectious diseases and emerging conditions. ICD-10 did not include these new diseases and disorders.

18.4.4 A Greater Degree of Particularity

ICD-11 provides increased specificity in coding, which makes it possible to convey diseases and conditions in a manner that is both precise and thorough. For accurate diagnosis and therapy, this level of specificity is very necessary.

18.4.5 Revisions Made to Chapters

The ICD-11 includes chapters that have been changed and reorganized to reflect changes in both medical knowledge and practices. These revisions result in a classification scheme that is both more comprehensive and up to date.

18.4.6 Utilization of Available Technology

ICD-11 takes advantage of technology to increase functionality, providing users with internet access and electronic tools to work with. Because of this, it is more suitable for use in contemporary medical environments.

18.4.7 User Interface Support for Multiple Languages

The ICD-11 can be obtained in a variety of tongues, which makes it approachable to users all around the world. This interface facilitates its application in a variety of healthcare settings thanks to its compatibility for multiple languages.

18.5 Methods of Implementation and Obstacles

The implementation of ICD-11 presents opportunities as well as obstacles for healthcare systems all across the world:

18.5.1 Difficulties in the Implementation

In order to prepare for the transfer to ICD-11, healthcare organizations need to upgrade their systems, train their employees, and guarantee that the accuracy of their coding is maintained throughout the shift.

18.5.2 The Consistency of the Data

For the sake of both patient treatment and insurance reimbursement, ensuring data consistency between ICD-10 and ICD-11 is essential. In order to avoid disruptions in both billing and patient treatment, healthcare providers need to carefully manage this shift.

18.5.3 Impact on the World

Because it is utilized on a global scale, the ICD-11 has an effect on healthcare practitioners, researchers, and public health agencies all over the world. The revisions it contains have the potential to improve healthcare all throughout the world.

18.5.4 An Increased Capability for Accuracy

Because of its increased specificity and terminology, ICD-11 presents the possibility of more accurate coding and, as a result, improved patient care.

18.6 The Clinical Modification of the International Classification of Diseases, 10th Revision (ICD-10-CM)

ICD-10-CM is a clinical variant of the ICD-10 system that is commonly used for diagnostic coding in the United States. In other words, ICD-10-CM is an abbreviation. The increased level of depth and precision offered by ICD-10-CM enables more accurate coding within the context of the healthcare system in the United States.

18.6.1 The Organization of the ICD-10-CM

The ICD-10-CM follows a framework that is very similar to that of the ICD-10, but it also incorporates codes and standards that are intended specifically for the healthcare system in the United States.

18.6.2 The Advantages of Using ICD-10-CM

ICD-10-CM provides a number of advantages, including greater precision in medical coding and billing, heightened awareness of and response to threats to public health, and enhanced facilitation of research and clinical decision-making.

18.6.3 Obstacles There Will Be

Because it was such a radical change from its predecessor, ICD-9-CM, the move from ICD-9-CM to ICD-10-CM in the United States required a large investment of time and resources on the part of healthcare organizations.

18.7 Upcoming Changes and Observations

It is anticipated that the ICD system will continue to develop in order to accommodate the shifting requirements of the healthcare environment:

18.7.1 Ongoing Upgrades and Patches

ICD-11 is not a fixed system, but rather one that will undergo constant modifications in order to keep up with developments in medical knowledge and new health concerns as they arise.

18.7.2 Integration with the Medical Technology and Information System

It is anticipated that the incorporation of ICD into health information technology systems will result in an improvement in both the accuracy and efficiency of data gathering and disease classification.

18.7.3 Cooperation on a Global Scale

Collaboration across international borders will continue to play an essential part in the expansion and upkeep of the ICD system, which will help to ensure that it remains relevant on a worldwide basis.

Practice Questions and Answers Explanations 2023-2024

Question 1
A patient receives a routine physical examination and is found to have high blood pressure. Which ICD-10-CM code should be used for the diagnosis of hypertension?
A) I10
B) I20
C) I30
D) I40

Answer 1
A) I10

Explanation 1
The ICD-10-CM code for essential (primary) hypertension is I10.

Question 2
Which of the following healthcare regulations in the United States prohibits healthcare providers from offering, paying, soliciting, or receiving remuneration for patient referrals?
A) HIPAA
B) Stark Law
C) ACA
D) OSHA

Answer 2
B) Stark Law

Explanation 2
Stark Law prohibits healthcare providers from offering, paying, soliciting, or receiving remuneration for patient referrals to entities with which the referring provider has a financial relationship.

Question 3

What type of examination involves the examination of tissues, organs, and cells to diagnose diseases and conditions?
A) Radiological examination
B) Endoscopic examination
C) Anatomic pathology examination
D) Genetic examination

Answer 3
C) Anatomic pathology examination

Explanation 3
Anatomic pathology involves the examination of tissues, organs, and cells to diagnose diseases and conditions.

Question 4

In medical coding, what does the acronym CPT stand for?
A) Current Procedural Terminology
B) Common Patient Treatment
C) Code for Patient Testing
D) Clinical Procedure Tracking

Answer 4
A) Current Procedural Terminology

Explanation 4
CPT stands for Current Procedural Terminology and is used for coding medical procedures and services.

Question 5

Which of the following ICD-11 updates offers greater specificity in disease coding?
A) Inclusion of new conditions
B) Enhanced terminology
C) Structured format
D) Multilingual interface

Answer 5
B) Enhanced terminology

Explanation 5
The enhanced terminology in ICD-11 offers greater specificity in disease coding, allowing for more accurate representation of diseases and conditions.

Question 6
What legal framework in the United States addresses the submission of false or fraudulent claims to federal healthcare programs such as Medicare and Medicaid?
A) Anti-Kickback Statute
B) Stark Law
C) False Claims Act
D) HIPAA

Answer 6
C) False Claims Act

Explanation 6
The False Claims Act addresses the submission of false or fraudulent claims to federal healthcare programs.

Question 7
Which organization is responsible for maintaining and updating the International Classification of Diseases (ICD)?
A) American Health Information Management Association (AHIMA)
B) American Academy of Professional Coders (AAPC)
C) World Health Organization (WHO)
D) Centers for Medicare and Medicaid Services (CMS)

Answer 7
C) World Health Organization (WHO)

Explanation 7
The World Health Organization (WHO) is responsible for maintaining and updating the International Classification of Diseases (ICD).

Question 8
What is the primary purpose of the ICD system?
A) Diagnosing patients
B) Medical billing and reimbursement
C) Public health research
D) Clinical decision-making

Answer 8
B) Medical billing and reimbursement

Explanation 8
The primary purpose of the ICD system is to assist in medical billing and reimbursement by providing standardized codes for diseases and conditions.

Question 9
A patient is diagnosed with a type of leukemia that was not previously included in ICD-10. Which ICD system is more likely to include this new diagnosis?
A) ICD-9
B) ICD-10
C) ICD-11
D) CPT

Answer 9
C) ICD-11

Explanation 9
ICD-11 includes new diseases and conditions that were not present in ICD-10, reflecting changes in the healthcare landscape.

Question 10
Which coding system is used for diagnostic coding in the United States and includes detailed codes and guidelines for American healthcare practices?
A) ICD-10-CM
B) ICD-11
C) CPT
D) ICD-10-PCS

Answer 10
A) ICD-10-CM

Explanation 10
ICD-10-CM is used for diagnostic coding in the United States and includes detailed codes and guidelines for American healthcare practices.

Question 11
A patient presents with severe chest pain. Which E/M code should be used for the evaluation and management of this patient in the emergency department?
A) 99201
B) 99203
C) 99205
D) 99213

Answer 11
C) 99205

Explanation 11
For a patient with severe chest pain in the emergency department, a higher-level E/M code like 99205 would be appropriate due to the complexity and severity of the condition.

Question 12
Which healthcare law focuses on safeguarding patients' protected health information (PHI)?
A) Stark Law
B) ACA
C) False Claims Act
D) HIPAA

Answer 12
D) HIPAA

Explanation 12
HIPAA (Health Insurance Portability and Accountability Act) focuses on safeguarding patients' protected health information (PHI).

Question 13

What is the primary purpose of ICD-11's structured format?

A) Enhancing clinical care

B) Facilitating data collection

C) Increasing coding complexity

D) Improving electronic health records

Answer 13

A) Enhancing clinical care

Explanation 13

ICD-11's structured format is designed to enhance clinical care by providing a user-friendly framework for disease classification.

Question 14

Which ICD-11 update is particularly important for global users and accessibility?

A) Inclusion of new conditions

B) Multilingual interface

C) Structured format

D) Enhanced terminology

Answer 14

B) Multilingual interface

Explanation 14

The multilingual interface in ICD-11 is important for global users, making it accessible in multiple languages.

Question 15

What type of examination involves the diagnosis and treatment of conditions related to the urinary system and male reproductive organs?

A) Radiological examination

B) Gynecological examination

C) Urological examination

D) Cardiac examination

Answer 15

C) Urological examination

Explanation 15
Urological examination involves the diagnosis and treatment of conditions related to the urinary system and male reproductive organs.

Question 16
In the context of medical billing and coding, what does E/M stand for?
A) Emergency Management
B) Evaluation and Management
C) Electronic Medical Records
D) Experimental Medicine

Answer 16
B) Evaluation and Management

Explanation 16
In the context of medical billing and coding, E/M stands for Evaluation and Management, referring to codes used for documenting patient encounters.

Question 17
Which ICD system is known for its clinical modification designed specifically for the United States?
A) ICD-11
B) ICD-10-CM
C) ICD-10-PCS
D) ICD-9

Answer 17
B) ICD-10-CM

Explanation 17
ICD-10-CM is known for its clinical modification designed specifically for the United States, providing detailed diagnostic codes.

Question 18
What is the primary function of the American Academy of Professional Coders (AAPC)?
A) Developing medical coding standards
B) Certifying medical coders
C) Regulating healthcare billing
D) Administering Medicaid

Answer 18
B) Certifying medical coders

Explanation 18
The primary function of the American Academy of Professional Coders (AAPC) is to certify medical coders.

Question 19
Which government agency oversees the administration of the Medicare and Medicaid programs in the United States?
A) CDC
B) FDA
C) CMS
D) WHO

Answer 19
C) CMS

Explanation 19
The Centers for Medicare and Medicaid Services (CMS) oversees the administration of the Medicare and Medicaid programs in the United States.

Question 20
A patient presents with a skin condition, and the healthcare provider is uncertain about the diagnosis. Which ICD-10-CM code is appropriate for an uncertain diagnosis?
A) NOS
B) NEC
C) NOS and NEC
D) Not billable

Answer 20
C) NOS and NEC

Explanation 20
In ICD-10-CM, "NOS" (Not Otherwise Specified) and "NEC" (Not Elsewhere Classified) codes are used for uncertain or unspecified diagnoses, allowing for billing in such cases.

Question 21

What type of examination involves the examination of the digestive system using a thin, flexible tube with a camera at the end?
A) Radiological examination
B) Endoscopic examination
C) Cardiac examination
D) Neurological examination

Answer 21
B) Endoscopic examination

Explanation 21
Endoscopic examination involves the examination of the digestive system using a thin, flexible tube with a camera at the end.

Question 22

Which of the following medical coding organizations emphasizes professional development, integrity, and confidentiality in its Code of Ethics?
A) CDC
B) CMS
C) AHIMA
D) WHO

Answer 22
C) AHIMA

Explanation 22
The American Health Information Management Association (AHIMA) emphasizes professional development, integrity, and confidentiality in its Code of Ethics for healthcare information management professionals.

Question 23

In the context of medical coding, what does CPT stand for?
A) Current Procedural Terminology
B) Clinical Pathology Testing
C) Coding and Patient Tracking
D) Clinical Procedure Technology

Answer 23
A) Current Procedural Terminology

Explanation 23
In the context of medical coding, CPT stands for Current Procedural Terminology, used for coding medical procedures and services.

Question 24
Which ICD system is known for its clinical modification designed specifically for inpatient procedure coding?
A) ICD-11
B) ICD-10-CM
C) ICD-10-PCS
D) ICD-9

Answer 24
C) ICD-10-PCS

Explanation 24
ICD-10-PCS is known for its clinical modification designed specifically for inpatient procedure coding.

Question 25
Which coding system is primarily used for documenting and billing medical procedures, surgeries, and interventions?
A) ICD-10-CM
B) CPT
C) ICD-10-PCS
D) ICD-11

Answer 25
B) CPT

Explanation 25
CPT (Current Procedural Terminology) is primarily used for documenting and billing medical procedures, surgeries, and interventions.

Question 26
A patient's healthcare provider prescribes a new medication, and the patient experiences a severe allergic reaction. Which ICD-10-CM code is appropriate for the diagnosis of an adverse effect of a drug or medication?
A) Z79.899
B) T88.7
C) L50.0
D) Y63.9

Answer 26
B) T88.7

Explanation 26
The ICD-10-CM code T88.7 is used for the diagnosis of an adverse effect of a drug or medication.

Question 27
Which of the following terms refers to the process of verifying a patient's insurance coverage before providing medical services?
A) Preauthorization
B) Post-claim review
C) Denial management
D) Concurrent review

Answer 27
A) Preauthorization

Explanation 27
Preauthorization is the process of verifying a patient's insurance coverage before providing medical services to ensure that the services will be covered.

Question 28
A patient's diagnosis includes the term "bilateral." What does this term indicate in medical coding?
A) The condition affects both sides of the body or a pair of organs.
B) The condition is not specific and requires further evaluation.
C) The condition is unrelated to the patient's primary complaint.
D) The patient is not responsive to treatment.

Answer 28

A) The condition affects both sides of the body or a pair of organs.

Explanation 28
In medical coding, "bilateral" indicates that the condition affects both sides of the body or a pair of organs.

Question 29
Which of the following CPT codes is typically used for a comprehensive office visit for a new patient?
A) 99201
B) 99212
C) 99203
D) 99215

Answer 29
C) 99203

Explanation 29
CPT code 99203 is typically used for a comprehensive office visit for a new patient with an expanded problem-focused history and examination.

Question 30
In ICD-10-CM, the term "sequela" is used to indicate what?
A) A secondary diagnosis resulting from the primary condition
B) A condition that is not yet diagnosed
C) A condition that is self-limiting and requires no treatment
D) A condition that is contagious

Answer 30
A) A secondary diagnosis resulting from the primary condition

Explanation 30
In ICD-10-CM, the term "sequela" is used to indicate a secondary diagnosis resulting from the primary condition, often referring to a condition that developed as a result of a previous injury or disease.

Question 31
Which of the following coding systems is primarily used for inpatient hospital procedures, surgeries, and interventions?
A) ICD-10-CM
B) CPT
C) ICD-11
D) ICD-10-PCS

Answer 31
D) ICD-10-PCS

Explanation 31
ICD-10-PCS is primarily used for inpatient hospital procedures, surgeries, and interventions.

Question 32
A patient's medical record includes the abbreviation "NOS" in the diagnosis section. What does "NOS" stand for in medical coding?
A) Not Otherwise Specified
B) Not Otherwise Suspected
C) New Onset Syndrome
D) No Other Symptoms

Answer 32
A) Not Otherwise Specified

Explanation 32
In medical coding, "NOS" stands for "Not Otherwise Specified" and is used when a diagnosis is not further specified.

Question 33
What type of examination involves the evaluation of a patient's central nervous system, including the brain and spinal cord?
A) Radiological examination
B) Neurological examination
C) Ophthalmological examination
D) Urological examination

Answer 33
B) Neurological examination

Explanation 33
A neurological examination involves the evaluation of a patient's central nervous system, including the brain and spinal cord.

Question 34
Which of the following organizations is responsible for maintaining and updating the ICD-10-CM system in the United States?
A) Centers for Medicare and Medicaid Services (CMS)
B) World Health Organization (WHO)
C) American Health Information Management Association (AHIMA)
D) American Academy of Professional Coders (AAPC)

Answer 34
A) Centers for Medicare and Medicaid Services (CMS)

Explanation 34
The Centers for Medicare and Medicaid Services (CMS) is responsible for maintaining and updating the ICD-10-CM system in the United States.

Question 35
In ICD-11, which update allows for improved electronic access and search capabilities?
A) Enhanced terminology
B) Inclusion of new conditions
C) Multilingual interface
D) Structured format

Answer 35
D) Structured format

Explanation 35
The structured format in ICD-11 allows for improved electronic access and search capabilities.

Question 36

A healthcare provider is performing a procedure on a patient, and the procedure is not found in the CPT code set. What action should the provider take?

A) Use an unspecified code.

B) Choose the code for a similar procedure.

C) Use a CPT modifier.

D) Contact the American Medical Association for a new code.

Answer 36

B) Choose the code for a similar procedure.

Explanation 36

When a procedure is not found in the CPT code set, the provider should choose the code for a similar procedure that best represents the service performed.

Question 37

What type of examination involves the examination of the female reproductive system?

A) Radiological examination

B) Gynecological examination

C) Ophthalmological examination

D) Endoscopic examination

Answer 37

B) Gynecological examination

Explanation 37

A gynecological examination involves the examination of the female reproductive system.

Question 38

In the context of medical coding, what does CCI stand for?

A) Correct Coding Initiative

B) Current Coding Index

C) Coding Compliance Indicator

D) Clinical Coding Instruction

Answer 38

A) Correct Coding Initiative

Explanation 38
In the context of medical coding, CCI stands for Correct Coding Initiative, a program that promotes accurate coding and reimbursement.

Question 39
Which coding system is primarily used for documenting and billing inpatient procedures in hospital settings?
A) ICD-10-CM
B) CPT
C) ICD-11
D) ICD-10-PCS

Answer 39
D) ICD-10-PCS

Explanation 39
ICD-10-PCS is primarily used for documenting and billing inpatient procedures in hospital settings.

Question 40
A patient presents with a deep cut on their hand that requires sutures. Which E/M code should be used for the evaluation and management of this patient's injury?
A) 99202
B) 99213
C) 99281
D) 99284

Answer 40
C) 99281

Explanation 40
For a patient with a simple injury like a deep cut on the hand that requires sutures, a lower-level E/M code like 99281 is appropriate.

Question 41

In the context of medical coding, what does "LCD" stand for?
A) Limited Coverage Determination
B) Local Coverage Determination
C) Longitudinal Coding Directive
D) Local Coding Directive

Answer 41
B) Local Coverage Determination

Explanation 41
In the context of medical coding, "LCD" stands for Local Coverage Determination, which provides information on coverage policies specific to a particular geographic area.

Question 42

Which of the following ICD-11 updates focuses on making the system more adaptable to modern healthcare settings?
A) Inclusion of new conditions
B) Structured format
C) Enhanced terminology
D) Use of technology

Answer 42
D) Use of technology

Explanation 42
The use of technology in ICD-11 focuses on making the system more adaptable to modern healthcare settings.

Question 43

A patient is diagnosed with an infectious disease. Which ICD-10-CM code should be used for the diagnosis of an infectious disease?
A) Z22.32
B) J96.00
C) R23.5
D) K58.9

Answer 43
B) J96.00

Explanation 43
ICD-10-CM codes beginning with "J" are used for diseases of the respiratory system, including infectious diseases.

Question 44
What organization is responsible for developing and maintaining the CPT code set?
A) American Health Information Management Association (AHIMA)
B) American Academy of Professional Coders (AAPC)
C) Centers for Medicare and Medicaid Services (CMS)
D) American Medical Association (AMA)

Answer 44
D) American Medical Association (AMA)

Explanation 44
The American Medical Association (AMA) is responsible for developing and maintaining the CPT code set.

Question 45
Which of the following is a key component of the revenue cycle in healthcare?
A) E/M coding
B) ICD-10-CM coding
C) Denial management
D) National Drug Code (NDC)

Answer 45
C) Denial management

Explanation 45
Denial management is a key component of the revenue cycle in healthcare, focusing on resolving claim denials to ensure timely reimbursement.

Question 46

In the United States, which government agency is responsible for regulating workplace safety in healthcare settings?
A) CDC
B) FDA
C) CMS
D) OSHA

Answer 46
D) OSHA

Explanation 46
The Occupational Safety and Health Administration (OSHA) is responsible for regulating workplace safety, including healthcare settings.

Question 47

A patient is diagnosed with a disorder affecting both the right and left kidneys. Which ICD-10-CM code should be used for this diagnosis?
A) N29.1
B) N25.0
C) N26.9
D) N26.1

Answer 47
B) N25.0

Explanation 47
ICD-10-CM code N25.0 is used for a disorder affecting both the right and left kidneys.

Question 48

What type of examination involves the evaluation of the heart and its function using techniques like echocardiography and electrocardiography?
A) Radiological examination
B) Gynecological examination
C) Cardiac examination
D) Ophthalmological examination

Answer 48
C) Cardiac examination

Explanation 48
A cardiac examination involves the evaluation of the heart and its function using techniques like echocardiography and electrocardiography.

Question 49
In medical coding, what does "NDC" stand for?
A) National Drug Code
B) National Diagnosis Code
C) Normal Diagnostic Classification
D) Non-Definitive Condition

Answer 49
A) National Drug Code

Explanation 49
In medical coding, "NDC" stands for National Drug Code, a unique identifier for prescription and over-the-counter medications.

Question 50
What is the primary purpose of ICD-10-PCS (Procedural Coding System)?
A) Documenting patient diagnoses
B) Classifying diseases and conditions
C) Coding inpatient hospital procedures
D) Coding outpatient medical procedures

Answer 50
C) Coding inpatient hospital procedures

Explanation 50
The primary purpose of ICD-10-PCS is to code inpatient hospital procedures in healthcare settings.

Question 51
Which of the following is a key component of medical billing?
A) ICD-10-PCS coding
B) Healthcare provider diagnosis
C) CPT coding
D) Patient's insurance card

Answer 51
C) CPT coding

Explanation 51
CPT coding is a key component of medical billing, as it represents the services and procedures provided to the patient.

Question 52
A patient is diagnosed with a rare genetic disorder that is not found in ICD-10-CM. Which coding system is more likely to include this new diagnosis?
A) ICD-9
B) ICD-10
C) ICD-11
D) CPT

Answer 52
C) ICD-11

Explanation 52
ICD-11 is more likely to include a new and rare diagnosis that was not present in ICD-10.

Question 53
Which of the following is an important consideration in the use of modifiers in medical coding?
A) Modifiers are used to increase reimbursement.
B) Modifiers are always numeric.
C) Modifiers are optional and can be omitted.
D) Modifiers provide additional information about a service or procedure.

Answer 53
D) Modifiers provide additional information about a service or procedure.

Explanation 53
Modifiers in medical coding provide additional information about a service or procedure, aiding in accurate billing and coding.

Question 54

A healthcare provider is performing a colonoscopy for both diagnostic and therapeutic purposes. Which modifier is commonly used in this situation to indicate both services?

A) -24

B) -25

C) -50

D) -59

Answer 54

D) -59

Explanation 54

Modifier -59 is commonly used to indicate that a procedure includes both diagnostic and therapeutic components.

Question 55

A patient's medical record includes the term "NOS" in the diagnosis section. What does "NOS" stand for in medical coding?

A) Not Otherwise Specified

B) No Other Symptoms

C) Not Otherwise Stated

D) Non-Operative Surgery

Answer 55

A) Not Otherwise Specified

Explanation 55

In medical coding, "NOS" stands for "Not Otherwise Specified," indicating that the diagnosis is not further specified.

Question 56

What is the primary purpose of the National Drug Code (NDC) system in medical billing and coding?

A) Documenting patient diagnoses

B) Identifying healthcare providers

C) Coding medical procedures

D) Identifying prescription medications

Answer 56

D) Identifying prescription medications

Explanation 56
The primary purpose of the National Drug Code (NDC) system is to identify prescription and over-the-counter medications for billing and tracking purposes.

Question 57
Which of the following is a key component of the revenue cycle in healthcare?
A) E/M coding
B) ICD-10-CM coding
C) Denial management
D) National Drug Code (NDC)

Answer 57
C) Denial management

Explanation 57
Denial management is a key component of the revenue cycle in healthcare, focusing on resolving claim denials to ensure timely reimbursement.

Question 58
What organization is responsible for developing and maintaining the CPT code set?
A) American Health Information Management Association (AHIMA)
B) American Academy of Professional Coders (AAPC)
C) Centers for Medicare and Medicaid Services (CMS)
D) American Medical Association (AMA)

Answer 58
D) American Medical Association (AMA)

Explanation 58
The American Medical Association (AMA) is responsible for developing and maintaining the CPT code set.

Question 59

In the United States, which government agency is responsible for regulating workplace safety in healthcare settings?

A) CDC

B) FDA

C) CMS

D) OSHA

Answer 59

D) OSHA

Explanation 59

The Occupational Safety and Health Administration (OSHA) is responsible for regulating workplace safety, including healthcare settings.

Question 60

A patient is diagnosed with a disorder affecting both the right and left kidneys. Which ICD-10-CM code should be used for this diagnosis?

A) N29.1

B) N25.0

C) N26.9

D) N26.1

Answer 60

B) N25.0

Explanation 60

ICD-10-CM code N25.0 is used for a disorder affecting both the right and left kidneys.

Question 61

What is the primary purpose of ICD-10-PCS (Procedural Coding System)?

A) Documenting patient diagnoses

B) Classifying diseases and conditions

C) Coding inpatient hospital procedures

D) Coding outpatient medical procedures

Answer 61

C) Coding inpatient hospital procedures

Explanation 61
The primary purpose of ICD-10-PCS is to code inpatient hospital procedures in healthcare settings.

Question 62
Which of the following is a key component of medical billing?
A) ICD-10-PCS coding
B) Healthcare provider diagnosis
C) CPT coding
D) Patient's insurance card

Answer 62
C) CPT coding

Explanation 62
CPT coding is a key component of medical billing, as it represents the services and procedures provided to the patient.

Question 63
A patient is diagnosed with a rare genetic disorder that is not found in ICD-10-CM. Which coding system is more likely to include this new diagnosis?
A) ICD-9
B) ICD-10
C) ICD-11
D) CPT

Answer 63
C) ICD-11

Explanation 63
ICD-11 is more likely to include a new and rare diagnosis that was not present in ICD-10.

Question 64
Which of the following is an important consideration in the use of modifiers in medical coding?
A) Modifiers are used to increase reimbursement.
B) Modifiers are always numeric.
C) Modifiers are optional and can be omitted.
D) Modifiers provide additional information about a service or procedure.

Answer 64
D) Modifiers provide additional information about a service or procedure.

Explanation 64
Modifiers in medical coding provide additional information about a service or procedure, aiding in accurate billing and coding.

Question 65
A healthcare provider is performing a colonoscopy for both diagnostic and therapeutic purposes. Which modifier is commonly used in this situation to indicate both services?
A) -24
B) -25
C) -50
D) -59

Answer 65
D) -59

Explanation 65
Modifier -59 is commonly used to indicate that a procedure includes both diagnostic and therapeutic components.

Question 66
A patient's medical record includes the term "NOS" in the diagnosis section. What does "NOS" stand for in medical coding?
A) Not Otherwise Specified
B) No Other Symptoms
C) Not Otherwise Stated
D) Non-Operative Surgery

Answer 66
A) Not Otherwise Specified

Explanation 66
In medical coding, "NOS" stands for "Not Otherwise Specified," indicating that the diagnosis is not further specified.

Question 67

What is the primary purpose of the National Drug Code (NDC) system in medical billing and coding?
A) Documenting patient diagnoses
B) Identifying healthcare providers
C) Coding medical procedures
D) Identifying prescription medications

Answer 67
D) Identifying prescription medications

Explanation 67
The primary purpose of the National Drug Code (NDC) system is to identify prescription and over-the-counter medications for billing and tracking purposes.

Question 68

Which of the following is a key component of the revenue cycle in healthcare?
A) E/M coding
B) ICD-10-CM coding
C) Denial management
D) National Drug Code (NDC)

Answer 68
C) Denial management

Explanation 68
Denial management is a key component of the revenue cycle in healthcare, focusing on resolving claim denials to ensure timely reimbursement.

Question 69

What organization is responsible for developing and maintaining the CPT code set?
A) American Health Information Management Association (AHIMA)
B) American Academy of Professional Coders (AAPC)
C) Centers for Medicare and Medicaid Services (CMS)
D) American Medical Association (AMA)

Answer 69
D) American Medical Association (AMA)

Explanation 69
The American Medical Association (AMA) is responsible for developing and maintaining the CPT code set.

Question 70
In the United States, which government agency is responsible for regulating workplace safety in healthcare settings?
A) CDC
B) FDA
C) CMS
D) OSHA

Answer 70
D) OSHA

Explanation 70
The Occupational Safety and Health Administration (OSHA) is responsible for regulating workplace safety, including healthcare settings.

Question 71
A patient is diagnosed with a disorder affecting both the right and left kidneys. Which ICD-10-CM code should be used for this diagnosis?
A) N29.1
B) N25.0
C) N26.9
D) N26.1

Answer 71
B) N25.0

Explanation 71
ICD-10-CM code N25.0 is used for a disorder affecting both the right and left kidneys.

Question 72
What is the primary purpose of ICD-10-PCS (Procedural Coding System)?
A) Documenting patient diagnoses
B) Classifying diseases and conditions
C) Coding inpatient hospital procedures

D) Coding outpatient medical procedures

Answer 72
C) Coding inpatient hospital procedures

Explanation 72
The primary purpose of ICD-10-PCS is to code inpatient hospital procedures in healthcare settings.

Question 73
Which of the following is a key component of medical billing?
A) ICD-10-PCS coding
B) Healthcare provider diagnosis
C) CPT coding
D) Patient's insurance card

Answer 73
C) CPT coding

Explanation 73
CPT coding is a key component of medical billing, as it represents the services and procedures provided to the patient.

Question 74
A patient is diagnosed with a rare genetic disorder that is not found in ICD-10-CM. Which coding system is more likely to include this new diagnosis?
A) ICD-9
B) ICD-10
C) ICD-11
D) CPT

Answer 74
C) ICD-11

Explanation 74
ICD-11 is more likely to include a new and rare diagnosis that was not present in ICD-10.

Question 75
Which of the following is an important consideration in the use of modifiers in medical coding?
A) Modifiers are used to increase reimbursement.
B) Modifiers are always numeric.
C) Modifiers are optional and can be omitted.
D) Modifiers provide additional information about a service or procedure.

Answer 75
D) Modifiers provide additional information about a service or procedure.

Explanation 75
Modifiers in medical coding provide additional information about a service or procedure, aiding in accurate billing and coding.

Question 76
A healthcare provider is performing a colonoscopy for both diagnostic and therapeutic purposes. Which modifier is commonly used in this situation to indicate both services?
A) -24
B) -25
C) -50
D) -59

Answer 76
D) -59

Explanation 76
Modifier -59 is commonly used to indicate that a procedure includes both diagnostic and therapeutic components.

Question 77
A patient's medical record includes the term "NOS" in the diagnosis section. What does "NOS" stand for in medical coding?
A) Not Otherwise Specified
B) No Other Symptoms
C) Not Otherwise Stated
D) Non-Operative Surgery

Answer 77

A) Not Otherwise Specified

Explanation 77
In medical coding, "NOS" stands for "Not Otherwise Specified," indicating that the diagnosis is not further specified.

Question 78
What is the primary purpose of the National Drug Code (NDC) system in medical billing and coding?
A) Documenting patient diagnoses
B) Identifying healthcare providers
C) Coding medical procedures
D) Identifying prescription medications

Answer 78
D) Identifying prescription medications

Explanation 78
The primary purpose of the National Drug Code (NDC) system is to identify prescription and over-the-counter medications for billing and tracking purposes.

Question 79
Which of the following is a key component of the revenue cycle in healthcare?
A) E/M coding
B) ICD-10-CM coding
C) Denial management
D) National Drug Code (NDC)

Answer 79
C) Denial management

Explanation 79
Denial management is a key component of the revenue cycle in healthcare, focusing on resolving claim denials to ensure timely reimbursement.

Question 80

What organization is responsible for developing and maintaining the CPT code set?

A) American Health Information Management Association (AHIMA)
B) American Academy of Professional Coders (AAPC)
C) Centers for Medicare and Medicaid Services (CMS)
D) American Medical Association (AMA)

Answer 80
D) American Medical Association (AMA)

Explanation 80
The American Medical Association (AMA) is responsible for developing and maintaining the CPT code set.

Question 81

What does the abbreviation "E/M" stand for in the context of medical coding?

A) Evaluation and Management
B) Emergency Medicine
C) Electronic Medical Records
D) Extended Monitoring

Answer 81
A) Evaluation and Management

Explanation 81
In medical coding, "E/M" stands for Evaluation and Management, referring to the coding of services related to the assessment and management of patient conditions.

Question 82

In ICD-10-CM coding, what does the "X" placeholder represent in an alphanumeric code?

A) A placeholder for a numeric digit
B) A placeholder for a letter
C) A placeholder for a decimal point
D) A placeholder for a hyphen

Answer 82
A) A placeholder for a numeric digit

Explanation 82
In ICD-10-CM coding, the "X" is a placeholder used for a numeric digit, allowing for future expansion of the code set.

Question 83
Which of the following coding systems is used for reporting medical services provided in outpatient settings?
A) ICD-10-CM
B) CPT
C) ICD-11
D) ICD-10-PCS

Answer 83
B) CPT

Explanation 83
CPT (Current Procedural Terminology) is used for reporting medical services provided in outpatient settings.

Question 84
A patient has received a diagnosis of "benign" for a specific condition. In ICD-10-CM, which term is used to indicate a benign condition?
A) "Mal"
B) "Beni"
C) "NOS"
D) "Neoplasm"

Answer 84
D) "Neoplasm"

Explanation 84
In ICD-10-CM, the term "Neoplasm" is used to indicate a benign condition.

Question 85
What is the purpose of the CPT modifier "-51"?
A) To indicate multiple procedures
B) To indicate a repeat procedure on the same day
C) To indicate a bilateral procedure
D) To indicate a discontinued procedure

Answer 85
A) To indicate multiple procedures

Explanation 85
The CPT modifier "-51" is used to indicate multiple procedures performed during the same session.

Question 86
Which organization is responsible for the development and publication of the ICD-10-CM code set?
A) American Medical Association (AMA)
B) World Health Organization (WHO)
C) American Health Information Management Association (AHIMA)
D) Centers for Medicare and Medicaid Services (CMS)

Answer 86
D) Centers for Medicare and Medicaid Services (CMS)

Explanation 86
The Centers for Medicare and Medicaid Services (CMS) is responsible for the development and publication of the ICD-10-CM code set.

Question 87
In the context of ICD-10-CM coding, what does the abbreviation "NOS" stand for?
A) Not Otherwise Specified
B) Not Otherwise Stated
C) No Other Symptoms
D) Non-Operative Surgery

Answer 87
A) Not Otherwise Specified

Explanation 87
In ICD-10-CM coding, "NOS" stands for "Not Otherwise Specified," indicating that the diagnosis is not further specified.

Question 88

What is the primary purpose of the Healthcare Common Procedure Coding System (HCPCS)?

A) To classify diseases and conditions
B) To code inpatient hospital procedures
C) To document patient diagnoses
D) To code medical services and supplies

Answer 88

D) To code medical services and supplies

Explanation 88

The primary purpose of the Healthcare Common Procedure Coding System (HCPCS) is to code medical services and supplies.

Question 89

In medical billing, what is the primary role of a clearinghouse?

A) To provide patient care
B) To determine E/M codes
C) To process and transmit claims
D) To perform ICD-10-PCS coding

Answer 89

C) To process and transmit claims

Explanation 89

In medical billing, a clearinghouse processes and transmits claims to payers on behalf of healthcare providers.

Question 90

Which of the following is a key component of the revenue cycle in healthcare?

A) E/M coding
B) ICD-10-CM coding
C) Denial management
D) National Drug Code (NDC)

Answer 90

C) Denial management

Explanation 90

Denial management is a key component of the revenue cycle in healthcare, focusing on resolving claim denials to ensure timely reimbursement.

Question 91
What is the primary purpose of an E/M code in medical coding?
A) To indicate a diagnosis code
B) To identify a medical procedure
C) To classify diseases and conditions
D) To describe the level of evaluation and management services

Answer 91
D) To describe the level of evaluation and management services

Explanation 91
E/M codes in medical coding describe the level of evaluation and management services provided during a patient encounter.

Question 92
In medical billing, what does "EDI" stand for?
A) Electronic Diagnosis Interface
B) Electronic Data Interchange
C) Efficient Data Integration
D) Essential Documentation Information

Answer 92
B) Electronic Data Interchange

Explanation 92
In medical billing, "EDI" stands for Electronic Data Interchange, a method of electronically exchanging healthcare information.

Question 93
A patient presents with a common cold and is diagnosed with "Acute Nasopharyngitis." What ICD-10-CM code should be used for this diagnosis?
A) J00.0
B) R05
C) N76.0
D) L00

Answer 93

A) J00.0

Explanation 93
ICD-10-CM code J00.0 is used for "Acute Nasopharyngitis," commonly known as the common cold.

Question 94
What is the primary purpose of the National Provider Identifier (NPI) in healthcare?
A) To identify a patient's insurance coverage
B) To track medical supplies and equipment
C) To uniquely identify healthcare providers
D) To determine ICD-10-PCS codes

Answer 94
C) To uniquely identify healthcare providers

Explanation 94
The National Provider Identifier (NPI) is used to uniquely identify healthcare providers for billing and administrative purposes.

Question 95
Which organization is responsible for developing and maintaining the HCPCS Level II code set?
A) American Medical Association (AMA)
B) Centers for Medicare and Medicaid Services (CMS)
C) World Health Organization (WHO)
D) American Health Information Management Association (AHIMA)

Answer 95
B) Centers for Medicare and Medicaid Services (CMS)

Explanation 95
The Centers for Medicare and Medicaid Services (CMS) is responsible for developing and maintaining the HCPCS Level II code set.

Question 96
In ICD-10-CM coding, what is the purpose of the "7th character" in certain codes?
A) To indicate a secondary diagnosis

B) To specify the severity of an injury

C) To identify the patient's age

D) To differentiate between initial and subsequent encounters

Answer 96

D) To differentiate between initial and subsequent encounters

Explanation 96

In ICD-10-CM coding, the "7th character" is used to differentiate between initial and subsequent encounters for injuries and conditions.

Question 97

Which of the following is an example of an "external cause code" in ICD-10-CM?

A) S72.301A

B) W22.01XD

C) J45.902

D) N39.0

Answer 97

B) W22.01XD

Explanation 97

"External cause codes" in ICD-10-CM, such as W22.01XD, provide information about how an injury or condition occurred.

Question 98

A patient presents with a fractured wrist. Which type of code should be used to describe the specific bone involved in the fracture?

A) E-code

B) Diagnosis code

C) Place of occurrence code

D) External cause code

Answer 98

B) Diagnosis code

Explanation 98

To describe the specific bone involved in a fracture, a diagnosis code from the ICD-10-CM system should be used.

Question 99
What is the primary purpose of the ICD-10-PCS (Procedural Coding System)?
A) Documenting patient diagnoses
B) Classifying diseases and conditions
C) Coding outpatient medical procedures
D) Coding inpatient hospital procedures

Answer 99
D) Coding inpatient hospital procedures

Explanation 99
The primary purpose of ICD-10-PCS is to code inpatient hospital procedures in healthcare settings.

Question 100
A patient is diagnosed with a contagious disease caused by a virus. Which ICD-10-CM code should be used for the diagnosis of a viral disease?
A) A00-B99
B) C00-D49
C) J00-J99
D) Z00-Z99

Answer 100
A) A00-B99

Explanation 100
ICD-10-CM codes in the range A00-B99 are used for infectious and parasitic diseases, including viral diseases.

Question 101
What is the primary purpose of a "claim scrubber" in medical billing?
A) To remove denied claims
B) To submit claims to payers
C) To validate claims for accuracy
D) To generate patient statements

Answer 101
C) To validate claims for accuracy

Explanation 101
A "claim scrubber" is a tool used in medical billing to validate claims for accuracy before submission to payers.

Question 102
In the context of medical billing, what does the abbreviation "EOB" stand for?
A) Explanation of Benefits
B) Electronic Office Billing
C) Excessive Overhead Billing
D) Efficacy of Billing

Answer 102
A) Explanation of Benefits

Explanation 102
In medical billing, "EOB" stands for Explanation of Benefits, which is a statement sent by a payer to explain the processing of a claim.

Question 103
What type of code is found in the HCPCS Level II code set?
A) Diagnosis codes
B) Procedure codes
C) Place of occurrence codes
D) Supply codes

Answer 103
D) Supply codes

Explanation 103
The HCPCS Level II code set includes supply codes, which are used to identify medical supplies and equipment.

Question 104
A healthcare provider is performing a procedure that is not widely performed, and there is no specific CPT code available. What type of code should be used in this situation?
A) E/M code
B) Placeholder code
C) Unlisted procedure code
D) ICD-10-PCS code

Answer 104
C) Unlisted procedure code

Explanation 104
In cases where a specific CPT code is not available, an "unlisted procedure code" is used to describe the service provided.

Question 105
What does "EDI" stand for in the context of electronic claims processing?
A) Electronic Data Integration
B) Efficient Data Interface
C) Electronic Data Interchange
D) Exceptional Data Integration

Answer 105
C) Electronic Data Interchange

Explanation 105
In the context of electronic claims processing, "EDI" stands for Electronic Data Interchange, which is the electronic exchange of healthcare data.

Question 106
A patient has received a diagnosis of "Influenza due to unidentified influenza virus." Which ICD-10-CM code should be used for this diagnosis?
A) J09.X2
B) J10.0
C) J11.0
D) J14.1

Answer 106
A) J09.X2

Explanation 106
The code J09.X2 is used for "Influenza due to unidentified influenza virus."

Question 107

What is the primary purpose of a "Clean Claim" in medical billing?
A) To describe complex medical procedures
B) To submit a claim to a payer
C) To ensure accurate diagnosis coding
D) To have a claim without errors or deficiencies

Answer 107
D) To have a claim without errors or deficiencies

Explanation 107
A "Clean Claim" is a claim that is free of errors or deficiencies and can be processed by a payer without delays.

Question 108

Which organization is responsible for developing and maintaining the ICD-11 code set?
A) American Medical Association (AMA)
B) World Health Organization (WHO)
C) Centers for Medicare and Medicaid Services (CMS)
D) American Health Information Management Association (AHIMA)

Answer 108
B) World Health Organization (WHO)

Explanation 108
The World Health Organization (WHO) is responsible for developing and maintaining the ICD-11 code set.

Question 109

In the context of medical billing, what does "RVU" stand for?
A) Relative Value Unit
B) Reimbursement Verification Update
C) Reasonable and Customary Value
D) Relative Value Update

Answer 109
A) Relative Value Unit

Explanation 109

In medical billing, "RVU" stands for Relative Value Unit, which is used to determine the value of medical services for reimbursement.

Question 110
A patient has been diagnosed with a condition that affects the cardiovascular system. Which range of ICD-10-CM codes should be used for cardiovascular diseases?
A) C00-D49
B) I00-I99
C) N00-N99
D) S00-T88

Answer 110
B) I00-I99

Explanation 110
ICD-10-CM codes in the range I00-I99 are used for cardiovascular diseases and conditions.

Question 111
What is the primary purpose of a "Superbill" in medical billing?
A) To document patient diagnoses
B) To provide patient education
C) To code medical procedures
D) To capture services and charges

Answer 111
D) To capture services and charges

Explanation 111
A "Superbill" is used to capture the services and charges provided to a patient during a healthcare visit.

Question 112
In the context of medical billing, what is the purpose of the "ICD-10-CM Tabular List"?
A) To provide a detailed index of CPT codes
B) To list all valid ICD-10-CM diagnosis codes
C) To describe the reimbursement process
D) To define the structure of E/M codes

Answer 112
B) To list all valid ICD-10-CM diagnosis codes

Explanation 112
The "ICD-10-CM Tabular List" is a comprehensive list of all valid ICD-10-CM diagnosis codes.

Question 113
What is the primary purpose of the "CMS-1500" form in medical billing?
A) To record patient medical history
B) To document patient demographics
C) To submit claims to payers
D) To provide patient education

Answer 113
C) To submit claims to payers

Explanation 113
The "CMS-1500" form is used to submit healthcare claims to payers for reimbursement.

Question 114
A healthcare provider is performing a procedure that is not widely performed, and there is no specific CPT code available. What type of code should be used in this situation?
A) E/M code
B) Placeholder code
C) Unlisted procedure code
D) ICD-10-PCS code

Answer 114
C) Unlisted procedure code

Explanation 114
In cases where a specific CPT code is not available, an "unlisted procedure code" is used to describe the service provided.

Question 115

In medical billing, what is the purpose of a "charge description master" (CDM)?

A) To list patient demographics
B) To provide insurance information
C) To track medical supplies
D) To establish the prices for services and procedures

Answer 115

D) To establish the prices for services and procedures

Explanation 115

A "charge description master" (CDM) is used to establish the prices for services and procedures provided by a healthcare facility.

Question 116

What type of code is found in the CPT code set?

A) Diagnosis codes
B) Procedure codes
C) Place of occurrence codes
D) Supply codes

Answer 116

B) Procedure codes

Explanation 116

The CPT code set includes procedure codes used to describe medical services and procedures.

Question 117

A patient presents with an injury resulting from a fall on a wet floor. Which type of code should be used to describe the external cause of the injury?

A) E-code
B) Diagnosis code
C) Place of occurrence code
D) External cause code

Answer 117

A) E-code

Explanation 117
E-codes (external cause codes) are used to describe the external cause of injuries and accidents.

Question 118
In the context of medical coding, what does "HIPAA" stand for?
A) Health Insurance Portability and Accountability Act
B) Healthcare Information Processing and Accreditation Act
C) Health Insurance Processing and Authorization Act
D) Hospital Information Privacy and Administration Act

Answer 118
A) Health Insurance Portability and Accountability Act

Explanation 118
In the context of medical coding, "HIPAA" stands for the Health Insurance Portability and Accountability Act, which sets standards for the protection of patient health information.

Question 119
What is the primary purpose of a "Remittance Advice" (RA) in medical billing?
A) To bill patients for services
B) To explain the denial of a claim
C) To provide a detailed medical record
D) To verify a patient's insurance coverage

Answer 119
B) To explain the denial of a claim

Explanation 119
A "Remittance Advice" (RA) in medical billing provides information about the processing of a claim, including denials and explanations.

Question 120
In the context of medical billing, what is the purpose of a "Benefit Verification" process?
A) To review the patient's medical history
B) To confirm a patient's identity
C) To determine insurance coverage and benefits
D) To assess the patient's financial status

Answer 120

C) To determine insurance coverage and benefits

Explanation 120

The "Benefit Verification" process in medical billing is used to determine a patient's insurance coverage and benefits.

Question 121

In ICD-10-CM coding, what is the purpose of the "7th character" in the code for a malignancy?
A) To indicate the primary site of the malignancy
B) To specify the stage of the malignancy
C) To denote a family history of malignancies
D) To describe the histology of the malignancy

Answer 121

B) To specify the stage of the malignancy

Explanation 121

In ICD-10-CM coding for malignancies, the "7th character" is used to specify the stage of the malignancy.

Question 122

What is the primary purpose of a "Master Patient Index" (MPI) in healthcare?
A) To list all healthcare facilities in a region
B) To document patient demographics
C) To track the prices of medical procedures
D) To create a comprehensive list of all patients

Answer 122

B) To document patient demographics

Explanation 122

A "Master Patient Index" (MPI) in healthcare is used to document and maintain patient demographics and identification information.

Question 123

In the context of medical billing, what does "PPO" stand for?

A) Primary Provider Organization

B) Preferred Provider Organization

C) Patient Payment Option

D) Physician Practice Operations

Answer 123

B) Preferred Provider Organization

Explanation 123

In medical billing, "PPO" stands for Preferred Provider Organization, a type of health insurance plan.

Question 124

A patient has received a diagnosis of "Stage I Breast Cancer." In ICD-10-CM coding, which "7th character" should be used to indicate this stage?

A) A

B) D

C) M

D) X

Answer 124

A) A

Explanation 124

In ICD-10-CM coding for malignancies, the "7th character" "A" is used to indicate Stage I.

Question 125

What is the primary purpose of the "EOB Remark Codes" in medical billing?

A) To provide additional information about a procedure

B) To list all valid ICD-10-CM diagnosis codes

C) To explain the denial or adjustment of a claim

D) To describe the medical supplies and equipment used

Answer 125

C) To explain the denial or adjustment of a claim

Explanation 125

EOB Remark Codes in medical billing are used to explain the denial or adjustment of a claim, providing additional information.

Question 126
A patient presents with a documented allergic reaction to a medication. In ICD-10-CM coding, which code should be used to describe the allergic reaction?
A) T78.4
B) Z88.0
C) R10.0
D) E85.9

Answer 126
A) T78.4

Explanation 126
ICD-10-CM code T78.4 is used for allergic reactions to medications and biological substances.

Question 127
In the context of medical billing, what is the purpose of a "Superbill"?
A) To document patient demographics
B) To provide patient education
C) To code medical procedures
D) To capture services and charges

Answer 127
D) To capture services and charges

Explanation 127
A "Superbill" is used to capture the services and charges provided to a patient during a healthcare visit.

Question 128
What is the primary purpose of the "Universal Product Number" (UPN) in medical billing and coding?
A) To identify healthcare providers
B) To code medical procedures
C) To track medical supplies and equipment
D) To uniquely identify medical products and drugs

Answer 128
D) To uniquely identify medical products and drugs

Explanation 128
The Universal Product Number (UPN) is used to uniquely identify medical products and drugs for billing and tracking purposes.

Question 129
In medical billing, what is the purpose of "Preauthorization"?
A) To document patient demographics
B) To validate claim accuracy
C) To obtain approval for medical services
D) To explain the denial of a claim

Answer 129
C) To obtain approval for medical services

Explanation 129
In medical billing, "Preauthorization" is the process of obtaining approval from a payer for specific medical services before they are provided.

Question 130
What is the primary purpose of the "Medical Coding Manual" in medical billing and coding?
A) To explain the denial of a claim
B) To track medical supplies and equipment
C) To list all valid ICD-10-CM diagnosis codes
D) To provide guidelines for assigning diagnosis and procedure codes

Answer 130
D) To provide guidelines for assigning diagnosis and procedure codes

Explanation 130
A "Medical Coding Manual" provides guidelines and instructions for assigning diagnosis and procedure codes in medical coding.

.

Question 131
In medical billing, what does the abbreviation "EOC" stand for?
A) Explanation of Charges
B) Episode of Care
C) Evaluation of Claims
D) Electronic Office Communication

Answer 131
B) Episode of Care

Explanation 131
In medical billing, "EOC" stands for Episode of Care, which refers to a period of healthcare delivery to a patient.

Question 132
A patient is diagnosed with a fracture that does not involve displacement. Which ICD-10-CM code should be used for this diagnosis?
A) S62.00
B) S62.1
C) S62.110
D) S62.121

Answer 132
A) S62.00

Explanation 132
ICD-10-CM code S62.00 is used for a nondisplaced fracture of the radius and ulna at the wrist and hand level.

Question 133
What is the primary purpose of "Medical Necessity" in medical coding?
A) To describe the location of a healthcare facility
B) To determine the medical history of a patient
C) To justify the need for a medical service
D) To establish the cost of a procedure

Answer 133
C) To justify the need for a medical service

Explanation 133

"Medical Necessity" in medical coding refers to the justification of the need for a medical service or procedure based on clinical criteria.

Question 134
In medical billing, what does "UB-04" refer to?
A) A type of health insurance plan
B) A claim form used for hospital services
C) A CPT code used for surgeries
D) A modifier used for diagnostic procedures

Answer 134
B) A claim form used for hospital services

Explanation 134
The "UB-04" is a claim form used for billing hospital services and is also known as the CMS-1450 form.

Question 135
Which organization is responsible for developing and maintaining the CPT code set?
A) American Health Information Management Association (AHIMA)
B) American Academy of Professional Coders (AAPC)
C) Centers for Medicare and Medicaid Services (CMS)
D) American Medical Association (AMA)

Answer 135
D) American Medical Association (AMA)

Explanation 135
The American Medical Association (AMA) is responsible for developing and maintaining the CPT code set.

Question 136
What is the primary purpose of a "Local Coverage Determination" (LCD) in medical billing?
A) To establish national healthcare policies
B) To provide patient education
C) To define the scope of services for a particular region
D) To determine reimbursement rates for medical procedures

Answer 136

C) To define the scope of services for a particular region

Explanation 136

A "Local Coverage Determination" (LCD) in medical billing defines the scope of covered services for a specific geographic area.

Question 137

A patient is diagnosed with an injury caused by a motor vehicle accident. Which type of code should be used to describe the external cause of the injury?

A) E-code

B) Diagnosis code

C) Place of occurrence code

D) External cause code

Answer 137

A) E-code

Explanation 137

E-codes (external cause codes) are used to describe the external cause of injuries and accidents, including those related to motor vehicle accidents.

Question 138

In medical billing, what is the primary purpose of a "Clean Claim"?

A) To describe complex medical procedures

B) To submit claims to payers

C) To ensure accurate diagnosis coding

D) To have a claim without errors or deficiencies

Answer 138

D) To have a claim without errors or deficiencies

Explanation 138

A "Clean Claim" is a claim that is free of errors or deficiencies and can be processed by a payer without delays.

Question 139

What is the primary purpose of the "National Drug Code" (NDC) in medical billing and coding?

A) To identify healthcare providers

B) To code medical procedures

C) To track medical supplies and equipment

D) To uniquely identify prescription medications

Answer 139

D) To uniquely identify prescription medications

Explanation 139

The National Drug Code (NDC) is used to uniquely identify prescription and over-the-counter medications for billing and tracking.

Question 140

In ICD-10-CM coding, what does the abbreviation "NEC" stand for?

A) Not Elsewhere Classified

B) No Exception Code

C) New Encounter Code

D) Non-Excluded Condition

Answer 140

A) Not Elsewhere Classified

Explanation 140

In ICD-10-CM coding, "NEC" stands for "Not Elsewhere Classified," indicating a diagnosis that does not fit into a more specific category.

Question 141

What is the primary purpose of a "Provider Enrollment" process in medical billing?

A) To document patient demographics

B) To establish a list of medical codes

C) To verify the credentials of healthcare providers

D) To provide guidelines for assigning diagnosis codes

Answer 141

C) To verify the credentials of healthcare providers

Explanation 141
The "Provider Enrollment" process in medical billing is used to verify the credentials and qualifications of healthcare providers.

Question 142
In medical billing, what is the purpose of a "Superbill"?
A) To document patient demographics
B) To provide patient education
C) To code medical procedures
D) To capture services and charges

Answer 142
D) To capture services and charges

Explanation 142
A "Superbill" is used to capture the services and charges provided to a patient during a healthcare visit.

Question 143
A patient has received a diagnosis of "Acute Pharyngitis." What ICD-10-CM code should be used for this diagnosis?
A) J02.0
B) K21.9
C) M05.4
D) R22.9

Answer 143
A) J02.0

Explanation 143
ICD-10-CM code J02.0 is used for "Acute Pharyngitis."

Question 144
What is the primary purpose of a "Master Patient Index" (MPI) in healthcare?
A) To list all healthcare facilities in a region
B) To document patient demographics
C) To track the prices of medical procedures
D) To create a comprehensive list of all patients

Answer 144

D) To create a comprehensive list of all patients

Explanation 144
A "Master Patient Index" (MPI) in healthcare is used to create a comprehensive list of all patients associated with a healthcare facility.

Question 145
In the context of medical billing, what does "HMO" stand for?
A) Healthcare Management Organization
B) Health Maintenance Organization
C) Hospital Medical Operations
D) Healthcare Methodology Organization

Answer 145
B) Health Maintenance Organization

Explanation 145
In the context of medical billing, "HMO" stands for Health Maintenance Organization, a type of health insurance plan.

Question 146
A patient presents with symptoms of depression. In ICD-10-CM coding, which code range should be used for mental and behavioral disorders?
A) F00-F09
B) I00-I99
C) S00-T88
D) M00-M99

Answer 146
D) M00-M99

Explanation 146
ICD-10-CM codes in the range M00-M99 are used for mental and behavioral disorders.

Question 147
What is the primary purpose of "NCCI Edits" in medical coding?
A) To create a list of excluded procedures
B) To provide clinical guidelines for coding
C) To identify medical specialties

D) To prevent improper coding of services

Answer 147
D) To prevent improper coding of services

Explanation 147
NCCI Edits (National Correct Coding Initiative) are designed to prevent improper coding of services by identifying code combinations that should not be reported together.

Question 148
In the context of medical billing, what does "CMS" stand for?
A) Clinical Management System
B) Center for Medical Services
C) Centers for Medicare and Medicaid Services
D) Comprehensive Medical Solutions

Answer 148
C) Centers for Medicare and Medicaid Services

Explanation 148
In the context of medical billing, "CMS" stands for the Centers for Medicare and Medicaid Services, a federal agency responsible for healthcare programs.

Question 149
A patient has been diagnosed with "Chronic Obstructive Pulmonary Disease." Which ICD-10-CM code range should be used for respiratory diseases?
A) A00-B99
B) I00-I99
C) J00-J99
D) S00-T88

Answer 149
C) J00-J99

Explanation 149
ICD-10-CM codes in the range J00-J99 are used for respiratory diseases and conditions.

Question 150
What is the primary purpose of "Modifier 25" in CPT coding?
A) To indicate a bilateral procedure
B) To identify a repeat procedure on the same day
C) To denote a distinct procedural service
D) To specify the severity of an injury

Answer 150
C) To denote a distinct procedural service

Explanation 150
In CPT coding, "Modifier 25" is used to denote a distinct procedural service provided on the same day as an evaluation and management (E/M) service.

Question 151
In medical billing, what is the purpose of a "Charge Description Master" (CDM)?
A) To document patient demographics
B) To provide insurance information
C) To list the prices for services and procedures
D) To establish the prices for medical supplies

Answer 151
C) To list the prices for services and procedures

Explanation 151
A "Charge Description Master" (CDM) in medical billing lists the prices for services and procedures provided by a healthcare facility.

Question 152
What is the primary purpose of a "National Provider Identifier" (NPI) in healthcare?
A) To identify healthcare providers
B) To code medical procedures
C) To document patient demographics
D) To track medical supplies and equipment

Answer 152
A) To identify healthcare providers

Explanation 152
The National Provider Identifier (NPI) is used to uniquely identify healthcare providers for billing and administrative purposes.

Question 153
In ICD-10-CM coding, what is the primary purpose of "Excludes1" notes in the Tabular List?
A) To indicate codes that should never be used together
B) To provide additional information about a diagnosis
C) To identify codes that are commonly used together
D) To specify the timing of a procedure

Answer 153
A) To indicate codes that should never be used together

Explanation 153
"Excludes1" notes in the ICD-10-CM Tabular List indicate codes that should never be used together.

Question 154
What is the primary purpose of a "Benefit Verification" process in medical billing?
A) To review the patient's medical history
B) To confirm a patient's identity
C) To determine insurance coverage and benefits
D) To assess the patient's financial status

Answer 154
C) To determine insurance coverage and benefits

Explanation 154
The "Benefit Verification" process in medical billing is used to determine a patient's insurance coverage and benefits.

Question 155

A patient has been diagnosed with a "Right Occipital Intracranial Hemorrhage." What ICD-10-CM code should be used for this diagnosis?
A) I61.1
B) S06.1
C) M96.1
D) L72.1

Answer 155
A) I61.1

Explanation 155
ICD-10-CM code I61.1 is used for a "Right Occipital Intracranial Hemorrhage."

Question 156

In medical billing, what is the purpose of a "Claim Adjudication" process?
A) To submit claims to payers
B) To describe complex medical procedures
C) To review the patient's medical history
D) To validate claims for accuracy

Answer 156
D) To validate claims for accuracy

Explanation 156
"Claim Adjudication" in medical billing is the process of validating claims for accuracy and completeness before they are processed by payers.

Question 157

What is the primary purpose of "Place of Service (POS)" codes in medical billing?
A) To identify the patient's insurance coverage
B) To determine the location of a healthcare facility
C) To code medical procedures
D) To track medical supplies and equipment

Answer 157
B) To determine the location of a healthcare facility

Explanation 157

"Place of Service (POS)" codes in medical billing are used to specify the location where a healthcare service was provided.

Question 158
A patient has received a diagnosis of "Type 2 Diabetes Mellitus." Which ICD-10-CM code range should be used for endocrine and metabolic diseases?
A) C00-D49
B) I00-I99
C) E00-E89
D) S00-T88

Answer 158
C) E00-E89

Explanation 158
ICD-10-CM codes in the range E00-E89 are used for endocrine and metabolic diseases.

Question 159
In the context of medical coding, what does "CPT" stand for?
A) Clinical Procedure Terminology
B) Current Procedural Terminology
C) Comprehensive Patient Tracking
D) Clinical Practice Test

Answer 159
B) Current Procedural Terminology

Explanation 159
In the context of medical coding, "CPT" stands for Current Procedural Terminology, which is a standard code set for medical procedures.

Question 160

What is the primary purpose of the "RA" (Remittance Advice) Remark Codes in medical billing?

A) To explain the denial or adjustment of a claim

B) To list all valid ICD-10-CM diagnosis codes

C) To describe the medical supplies and equipment used

D) To validate claims for accuracy

Answer 160

A) To explain the denial or adjustment of a claim

Explanation 160

RA (Remittance Advice) Remark Codes in medical billing are used to explain the denial or adjustment of a claim, providing additional information.

Question 161

A patient presents with symptoms of a urinary tract infection. What ICD-10-CM code range should be used for genitourinary diseases?

A) A00-B99

B) I00-I99

C) N00-N99

D) S00-T88

Answer 161

C) N00-N99

Explanation 161

ICD-10-CM codes in the range N00-N99 are used for genitourinary diseases and conditions.

Question 162

In medical billing, what is the purpose of a "Clean Claim"?

A) To describe complex medical procedures

B) To submit claims to payers

C) To ensure accurate diagnosis coding

D) To have a claim without errors or deficiencies

Answer 162

D) To have a claim without errors or deficiencies

Explanation 162
A "Clean Claim" is a claim that is free of errors or deficiencies and can be processed by a payer without delays.

Question 163
What is the primary purpose of a "Charge Description Master" (CDM) in medical billing?
A) To list patient demographics
B) To provide insurance information
C) To track the prices of medical procedures
D) To establish the prices for services and procedures

Answer 163
D) To establish the prices for services and procedures

Explanation 163
A "Charge Description Master" (CDM) is used to establish the prices for services and procedures provided by a healthcare facility.

Question 164
A patient presents with an injury caused by a fall on a slippery floor. Which type of code should be used to describe the external cause of the injury?
A) E-code
B) Diagnosis code
C) Place of occurrence code
D) External cause code

Answer 164
A) E-code

Explanation 164
E-codes (external cause codes) are used to describe the external cause of injuries and accidents, including those related to falls.

Question 165
In medical billing, what is the purpose of a "National Drug Code" (NDC)?
A) To identify healthcare providers
B) To code medical procedures
C) To document patient demographics
D) To uniquely identify prescription medications

Answer 165
D) To uniquely identify prescription medications

Explanation 165
The National Drug Code (NDC) is used to uniquely identify prescription and over-the-counter medications for billing and tracking.

Question 166
A patient has been diagnosed with "Acute Respiratory Failure." Which ICD-10-CM code range should be used for respiratory diseases?
A) A00-B99
B) I00-I99
C) J00-J99
D) S00-T88

Answer 166
C) J00-J99

Explanation 166
ICD-10-CM codes in the range J00-J99 are used for respiratory diseases and conditions.

Question 167
What is the primary purpose of "Modifier 59" in CPT coding?
A) To indicate a bilateral procedure
B) To identify a repeat procedure on the same day
C) To specify the severity of an injury
D) To denote a distinct procedural service

Answer 167
B) To identify a repeat procedure on the same day

Explanation 167
In CPT coding, "Modifier 59" is used to identify a repeat procedure that is distinct from other procedures performed on the same day.

Question 168

In medical billing, what is the purpose of a "National Coverage Determination" (NCD)?

A) To define the scope of services for a particular region

B) To establish national healthcare policies

C) To provide patient education

D) To determine reimbursement rates for medical procedures

Answer 168

B) To establish national healthcare policies

Explanation 168

A "National Coverage Determination" (NCD) in medical billing is used to establish national healthcare policies regarding the coverage of specific services.

Question 169

What is the primary purpose of "Modifier 26" in CPT coding?

A) To indicate a bilateral procedure

B) To identify a repeat procedure on the same day

C) To denote a distinct procedural service

D) To specify the technical component of a procedure

Answer 169

D) To specify the technical component of a procedure

Explanation 169

In CPT coding, "Modifier 26" is used to specify that only the professional component of a procedure is being billed.

Question 170

In the context of medical coding, what does "DRG" stand for?

A) Diagnostic Revenue Group

B) Disease-Related Group

C) Diagnosis and Reporting Group

D) Doctor-Related Guidance

Answer 170

B) Disease-Related Group

Explanation 170
In the context of medical coding, "DRG" stands for Disease-Related Group, which is used in the classification of inpatient hospital cases for reimbursement.

Question 171
What is the primary purpose of a "Superbill" in medical billing?
A) To document patient diagnoses
B) To provide patient education
C) To code medical procedures
D) To capture services and charges

Answer 171
D) To capture services and charges

Explanation 171
A "Superbill" is used to capture the services and charges provided to a patient during a healthcare visit.

Question 172
A patient is diagnosed with "Chronic Obstructive Pulmonary Disease." Which ICD-10-CM code range should be used for respiratory diseases?
A) A00-B99
B) I00-I99
C) J00-J99
D) S00-T88

Answer 172
C) J00-J99

Explanation 172
ICD-10-CM codes in the range J00-J99 are used for respiratory diseases and conditions.

Question 173
In the context of medical billing, what does "PPO" stand for?
A) Primary Provider Organization
B) Preferred Provider Organization
C) Patient Payment Option
D) Physician Practice Operations

Answer 173
B) Preferred Provider Organization

Explanation 173
In medical billing, "PPO" stands for Preferred Provider Organization, a type of health insurance plan.

Question 174
What is the primary purpose of the "EOB Remark Codes" in medical billing?
A) To provide additional information about a procedure
B) To list all valid ICD-10-CM diagnosis codes
C) To explain the denial or adjustment of a claim
D) To describe the medical supplies and equipment used

Answer 174
C) To explain the denial or adjustment of a claim

Explanation 174
EOB Remark Codes in medical billing are used to explain the denial or adjustment of a claim, providing additional information.

Question 175
A patient presents with symptoms of a bacterial infection. What ICD-10-CM code range should be used for infectious and parasitic diseases?
A) A00-B99
B) I00-I99
C) J00-J99
D) S00-T88

Answer 175
A) A00-B99

Explanation 175
ICD-10-CM codes in the range A00-B99 are used for infectious and parasitic diseases.

Question 176

What is the primary purpose of a "Remittance Advice" (RA) in medical billing?

A) To bill patients for services

B) To explain the denial of a claim

C) To provide a detailed medical record

D) To verify a patient's insurance coverage

Answer 176

B) To explain the denial of a claim

Explanation 176

The "Remittance Advice" (RA) in medical billing provides information about the processing of a claim, including denials and explanations.

Question 177

A patient has been diagnosed with "Type 1 Diabetes Mellitus." Which ICD-10-CM code range should be used for endocrine and metabolic diseases?

A) C00-D49

B) I00-I99

C) E00-E89

D) S00-T88

Answer 177

C) E00-E89

Explanation 177

ICD-10-CM codes in the range E00-E89 are used for endocrine and metabolic diseases.

Question 178

In medical billing, what is the purpose of a "Clean Claim"?

A) To describe complex medical procedures

B) To submit claims to payers

C) To ensure accurate diagnosis coding

D) To have a claim without errors or deficiencies

Answer 178

D) To have a claim without errors or deficiencies

Explanation 178
A "Clean Claim" is a claim that is free of errors or deficiencies and can be processed by a payer without delays.

Question 179
What is the primary purpose of "Modifier 59" in CPT coding?
A) To indicate a bilateral procedure
B) To identify a repeat procedure on the same day
C) To specify the severity of an injury
D) To denote a distinct procedural service

Answer 179
B) To identify a repeat procedure on the same day

Explanation 179
In CPT coding, "Modifier 59" is used to identify a repeat procedure that is distinct from other procedures performed on the same day.

Question 180
In medical billing, what does "CMS" stand for?
A) Clinical Management System
B) Center for Medical Services
C) Centers for Medicare and Medicaid Services
D) Comprehensive Medical Solutions

Answer 180
C) Centers for Medicare and Medicaid Services

Explanation 180
In the context of medical billing, "CMS" stands for the Centers for Medicare and Medicaid Services, a federal agency responsible for healthcare programs.

Question 181
A patient has been diagnosed with "Hypertensive Heart Disease." What ICD-10-CM code should be used for this diagnosis?
A) I11.9
B) R99.9
C) L40.9
D) J98.9

Answer 181
A) I11.9

Explanation 181
ICD-10-CM code I11.9 is used for "Hypertensive Heart Disease."

Question 182
What is the primary purpose of a "National Provider Identifier" (NPI) in healthcare?
A) To identify healthcare providers
B) To code medical procedures
C) To document patient demographics
D) To track medical supplies and equipment

Answer 182
A) To identify healthcare providers

Explanation 182
The National Provider Identifier (NPI) is used to uniquely identify healthcare providers for billing and administrative purposes.

Question 183
In ICD-10-CM coding, what does the abbreviation "NOS" stand for?
A) Not Otherwise Specified
B) New Onset Symptoms
C) Normal Operating Standard
D) Non-Operative System

Answer 183
A) Not Otherwise Specified

Explanation 183
In ICD-10-CM coding, "NOS" stands for "Not Otherwise Specified," indicating that the diagnosis is not more specifically defined.

Question 184

What is the primary purpose of "Place of Service (POS)" codes in medical billing?

A) To identify the patient's insurance coverage
B) To determine the location of a healthcare facility
C) To code medical procedures
D) To track medical supplies and equipment .

Answer 184
B) To determine the location of a healthcare facility

Explanation 184
"Place of Service (POS)" codes in medical billing are used to specify the location where a healthcare service was provided.

Question 185

A patient has received a diagnosis of "Major Depressive Disorder." What ICD-10-CM code should be used for this diagnosis?

A) F32.9
B) I73.9
C) M51.9
D) R64.9

Answer 185
A) F32.9

Explanation 185
ICD-10-CM code F32.9 is used for "Major Depressive Disorder."

Question 186

In medical billing, what is the primary purpose of "Coordination of Benefits" (COB)?

A) To explain the denial of a claim
B) To document patient demographics
C) To determine the primary and secondary insurance coverage
D) To provide guidelines for assigning diagnosis codes

Answer 186
C) To determine the primary and secondary insurance coverage

Explanation 186
"Coordination of Benefits" (COB) in medical billing is the process of determining the primary and secondary insurance coverage for a patient.

Question 187
What is the primary purpose of "Modifier 26" in CPT coding?
A) To indicate a bilateral procedure
B) To identify a repeat procedure on the same day
C) To denote a distinct procedural service
D) To specify the technical component of a procedure

Answer 187
D) To specify the technical component of a procedure

Explanation 187
In CPT coding, "Modifier 26" is used to specify that only the professional component of a procedure is being billed.

Question 188
In the context of medical billing, what does "HMO" stand for?
A) Healthcare Management Organization
B) Health Maintenance Organization
C) Hospital Medical Operations
D) Healthcare Methodology Organization

Answer 188
B) Health Maintenance Organization

Explanation 188
In the context of medical billing, "HMO" stands for Health Maintenance Organization, a type of health insurance plan.

Question 189

A patient has been diagnosed with "Type 2 Diabetes Mellitus." What ICD-10-CM code should be used for this diagnosis?

A) I10

B) E11.9

C) M23.9

D) R57.9

Answer 189

B) E11.9

Explanation 189

ICD-10-CM code E11.9 is used for "Type 2 Diabetes Mellitus."

Question 190

What is the primary purpose of "Place of Service (POS)" codes in medical billing?

A) To identify the patient's insurance coverage

B) To determine the location of a healthcare facility

C) To code medical procedures

D) To track medical supplies and equipment

Answer 190

B) To determine the location of a healthcare facility

Explanation 190

"Place of Service (POS)" codes in medical billing are used to specify the location where a healthcare service was provided.

Question 191

In the context of medical coding, what does "ICD" stand for?

A) International Classification of Diseases

B) Inpatient Care Documentation

C) Internal Coding Directory

D) Insurance Claims Data

Answer 191

A) International Classification of Diseases

Explanation 191

In the context of medical coding, "ICD" stands for the International Classification of Diseases, which is used to code diagnoses and medical conditions.

Question 192
A patient has been diagnosed with "Acute Appendicitis." What ICD-10-CM code should be used for this diagnosis?
A) K35.9
B) S82.9
C) N10.9
D) T14.9

Answer 192
A) K35.9

Explanation 192
ICD-10-CM code K35.9 is used for "Acute Appendicitis."

Question 193
What is the primary purpose of "National Drug Code" (NDC) numbers in medical billing and coding?
A) To identify healthcare providers
B) To code medical procedures
C) To document patient demographics
D) To uniquely identify medical products and drugs

Answer 193
D) To uniquely identify medical products and drugs

Explanation 193
National Drug Code (NDC) numbers are used in medical billing and coding to uniquely identify medical products and drugs.

Question 194
In ICD-10-CM coding, what is the primary purpose of "Excludes2" notes in the Tabular List?
A) To indicate codes that should never be used together
B) To provide additional information about a diagnosis
C) To identify codes that are commonly used together
D) To specify the timing of a procedure

Answer 194

C) To identify codes that are commonly used together

Explanation 194

"Excludes2" notes in the ICD-10-CM Tabular List indicate codes that are commonly used together.

Question 195

What is the primary purpose of a "Charge Description Master" (CDM) in medical billing?

A) To list patient demographics

B) To provide insurance information

C) To track the prices of medical procedures

D) To establish the prices for medical supplies

Answer 195

C) To track the prices of medical procedures

Explanation 195

A "Charge Description Master" (CDM) in medical billing tracks the prices of medical procedures provided by a healthcare facility.

Question 196

A patient presents with symptoms of a skin rash. What ICD-10-CM code range should be used for skin and subcutaneous tissue diseases?

A) A00-B99

B) I00-I99

C) L00-L99

D) S00-T88

Answer 196

C) L00-L99

Explanation 196

ICD-10-CM codes in the range L00-L99 are used for skin and subcutaneous tissue diseases.

Question 197

In medical billing, what is the primary purpose of a "Clean Claim"?
A) To describe complex medical procedures
B) To submit claims to payers
C) To ensure accurate diagnosis coding
D) To have a claim without errors or deficiencies

Answer 197
D) To have a claim without errors or deficiencies

Explanation 197
A "Clean Claim" is a claim that is free of errors or deficiencies and can be processed by a payer without delays.

Question 198

What is the primary purpose of "Modifier 51" in CPT coding?
A) To indicate a bilateral procedure
B) To identify a repeat procedure on the same day
C) To specify the severity of an injury
D) To indicate multiple procedures performed during the same session

Answer 198
D) To indicate multiple procedures performed during the same session

Explanation 198
In CPT coding, "Modifier 51" is used to indicate that multiple procedures were performed during the same operative session.

Question 199

In the context of medical billing, what does "PPO" stand for?
A) Primary Provider Organization
B) Preferred Provider Organization
C) Patient Payment Option
D) Physician Practice Operations

Answer 199
B) Preferred Provider Organization

Explanation 199

In the context of medical billing, "PPO" stands for Preferred Provider Organization, a type of health insurance plan.

Question 200

A patient has been diagnosed with "Essential Hypertension." What ICD-10-CM code should be used for this diagnosis?
A) I10
B) J30.9
C) M42.9
D) L58.9

Answer 200
A) I10

Explanation 200
ICD-10-CM code I10 is used for "Essential Hypertension."